REVISED & UPDATED

The Odyssey of a Doctor Who Reversed
Fibromyalgia, Leaky Gut Syndrome &
Multiple Allergic Responses, NATURALLY...
...and Her Life 10 Years After Recovery

I was *Poisoned* by my body...

I have a gut feeling you could be, too!

Gloria Gilbère, N.D., D.A.Hom., Ph.D.
Foreword by Merry Alto, M.D.

Lucky
Press

ISBN: 978-0-9776300-6-6

Lucky Press, LLC
126 South Maple St., Lancaster, OH 43130
(740) 689-2950
Publisher's website: www.luckypress.com/gilbere
Publisher's email: books@luckypress.com

Author's website: www.gloriagilbere.com

Printed in the United States of America on elemental chlorine-free paper with soy-based inks.

Book design: Bonnie Lambert
Illustrations: Tama Bergstrand, Beata Golau, Bonnie Lambert
Dental photograph: Phil Gervais, D.D.S.

Library of Congress Cataloging-in-Publication Data

Gilbere, Gloria.
    I was poisoned by my body—I have a gut feeling you could be, too! : the
odyssey of a doctor who reversed fibromyalgia, leaky gut syndrome, multiple
allergic responses, naturally and her life 10 years after recovery / Gloria Gilbère;
foreword by Merry Alto.— 2nd ed.
        p. cm.
    ISBN-13: 978-0-9776300-6-6 (trade pbk. : alk. paper)
    1. Intestines—Diseases—Alternative treatment. 2. Gastrointestinal
system—Diseases—Alternative treatment. 3. Multiple chemical
sensitivity—Alternative treatment. 4. Autoimmune diseases—Alternative
treatment. 5. Environmentally induced diseases—Alternative treatment.
6. Naturopathy. I. Title.
    RC806.G55 2007
    362.196'340092--dc22
    [B]
                                2006102037

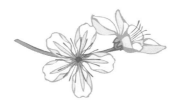

This book is dedicated to:

Muffy (a silver schnauzer) and her mother (Sharon), who made this book possible and taught me, by example, the true meaning of "unconditional love."

*The loving memory of my paternal grandmother…
my first "natural healer."*

*You, the reader, for taking this step
in pursuing natural health-care.*

Practitioners of the healing arts and pioneering physicians who have the unprejudiced and inquiring minds to search for fundamental causes of disease and drug-free therapies and, when found, the courage to proclaim and offer them for the benefit of their patients…even when the healing modality is contrary to currently accepted conventional consciousness and practices.

The thousands of loyal clients, readers, and students who have allowed me to be their health architect—following my design protocols on which to build a strong structure of wellness. I offer the blueprint—the building is to your credit. Your support facilitated the transformation of my life-threatening challenges into a professional service to assist those whose quality of life was robbed by invisible disorders as mine was.

To my creator, who facilitated my recovery and continues to be my strength. My prayer is that through my counsel, and this book, I continue to pave the way to health for all those willing to take the journey, Naturally.

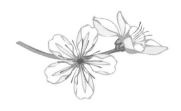

Important Author Update

WITH THIS UPDATED RELEASE, first published in 2000, it's important to keep in mind that the recommendations and therapies mentioned within are to be used as guidelines—every case is unique. After guiding thousands of clients around the world to wellness, experience proves what works and what doesn't.

Since my recovery from the disorders discussed within, many new products and healing modalities have come to light and are included in this edition.

Ten years after...I was POISONED by my body...

Many clients and readers ask if I have fully recovered. When you consider my current lifestyle, YOU DECIDE!

I...

- authored 8 books since the first printing of this book—*Invisible Illnesses*; *Nature's Prescription Milk*; *Pain/Inflammation Matters*; *Colon Cleansing Matters*; *Wholistic Skin & Body Rejuvenation*;

Healthy Travel Matters; CAM Skin Intensive; Silver Hydrosol

- maintain a worldwide private practice via telephone and my office in Idaho
- host a weekly talk-show "Your Health Matters" aired on www.healthylife.net
- wrote over 400 articles for health magazines and trade journals
- travel an average of 14 trips per year to lecture, teach and trade conferences
- completely remodeled a 20-year-old-home with all "safe" materials
- sit on the board of directors/advisors of several health organizations
- am adjunct faculty at Clayton College of Natural Health
- consult for product development for nutraceutical and cosmeceutical companies
- design, teach and guide individual programs for wholistic skin and body rejuvenation
- conduct health education and rejuvenation travel programs at destinations worldwide
- created my own rejuvenation skin care line—particularly for hypersensitive individuals

Do I live a "normal" life without limitations? That depends on your perspective of "normal." **I do not consume nightshade foods** because they induce inflammation; **I avoid toxic situations** (fragrances, pesticides, smoke, mold, etc.); **I protect my immune system** with silver hydrosol instead of antibiotics; **I no longer wear a mask**, yet always carry one; **I eat in restaurants** with attention to ingredient details, avoiding preservatives, flavor enhancers, coloring, etc.; **I live what I teach** and maintain detoxification protocols; **I enjoy life, giving thanks every day** that I was able to reverse the devastating health challenges into which I was thrust; **I give back** by validating victims of invisible illnesses, and by **designing protocols** for them to repair, and rebuild their health, *Naturally*.

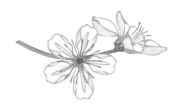

Contents

I was

Poisoned

by my body...

14

I was

Poisoned

by my body...

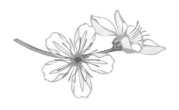

Foreword

1997—Merry Alto, M.D.

IT IS HUMBLING to have a patient with devastating illness, and despite all the years of education and training, be helpless in finding the cause and treatment for the illness.

It was almost one year ago when the author of this book—a highly educated and experienced alternative medicine professional—came to me with near anaphylactic-like allergic reactions to nearly all foods, hair loss, insomnia, myalgias, arthralgias, and profound fatigue. No test I did elucidated the cause. No treatment I gave helped and, in fact, only compounded the problem.

Dr. Gilbere researched her problem from the alternative medicine viewpoint and began treatment. Within a few weeks, the hair loss stopped and within a few months she looked healthier than I had ever seen her. The results were incontrovertible! I was astounded!

Fortunately, we do not see each other's educations and treatments at odds with each other, but rather quite complimentary—

each contributing something valuable to the care of our patients.

Please read Dr. Gilbere's personal case report; I can verify her remarkable results and encourage both mainstream and alternative medicine professionals to consider the leaky gut syndrome when faced with a baffling complex of patients.

—*Merry Alto, M.D.*

President, Washington State College
of Emergency Physicians
American Association of Physician Specialists
Association of Emergency Physicians
American College of Emergency Physicians

1997—Lola V. Righton, D.A.Hom.

IMAGE THIS: One day you're living a normal life, in a fulfilling profession you love, assisting others to live healthier, and doing so in a location that you specifically chose for its quality of life. Suddenly, everything in your world turns against you, and familiar surroundings and foods all cause a violent reaction several times a day—your face and neck turn beet red, your throat swells, and you can't swallow or breathe.

The following "ordinary" experiences literally threaten your life: every morsel of food you put in your mouth, the odor of every passing vehicle on the street, walking down the aisles in the grocery store, the chemical smells of furnishings and clothing, familiar items in your home and office, personal care and cleaning products you've used for years, fueling your car, entering a beauty shop, dental or medical facility, even going to your place of worship—each response triggering a violent reaction over which you have absolutely no control.

Multiple chemical sensitivities (MCS) are conditions triggered by our industrialized modern times. It affects all of us, even those who don't manifest the violent responses as Gloria did. In her practice, she has successfully assisted victims of invisible illnesses to wellness—the "canaries" in our society who are affected by toxic elements before others even validate their existence.

The complexity of MCS touches each of our lives, whether we admit or connect it or not. The effects of a ravaged immune system then causes severe nutritional deficiencies, digestive breakdown, and erosion of the protective mucosal coating of the intestines. Trashy particles of fecal matter and/or undigested proteins are absorbed directly into the blood supply causing a condition known as auto-intoxication or "leaky gut." Viewed under a microscope, your blood would look like a sewer…it is. No wonder you feel so awful.

Too many of us, when ill, rush to the medical community and lay ourselves at their feet saying, "Here I am, heal me," instead of taking responsibility for our health.

The answers are not solely found in printouts of laboratory analysis or expensive pieces of equipment interpreted by those trained in their small sphere of conventional application.

Health encompasses complex issues—success is not instantaneous, the road is arduous, physically and emotionally painful. Regaining health requires personal commitment, professional guidance, and perseverance.

It takes courage to pick up the unraveled strands of what is left of your health, discover the tools you need to begin knitting them back together, and then create and evolve your own instruction book. Gloria has done just that. It wasn't to impress anyone. It was to save a life; her own.

We have been colleagues in the field of alternative medicine for many years and have consulted on the more thorny problems of our clients and shared details of each other's health challenges—my health challenges started years ago, hers after a life-threatening accident and the repercussions of prescription medications.

After returning from what had promised to be a relaxing extended weekend, Gloria called me in great pain under her right breast and between her shoulders. After discussing her symptoms, we came to no conclusions as to an obvious cause, or for the persistent and debilitating effects on her life and ability to continue her holistic practice.

In the following pages, she recounts her increasingly desperate search for relief from the relentless, piercing pain, the consequences of conventional medical treatment, and her struggle to survive.

There is a terrible emotional toll on the sufferers of "leaky gut" and its related syndromes. Many of you are without support from physicians, family and friends who simply do not understand how someone who looks so "normal" from the outside can be in such misery. Your symptoms are often varied and seem unconnected by any conventional view yet, in fact, have a root cause.

It can be very lonely wondering if and, as you are no doubt sick of hearing, "It's all in your head." Reading this book will be of tremendous value and validation. You are NOT alone and you are NOT a "head" case, or as Gloria, respectfully referred to by her clients as "Dr. G", says, "You are not suffering from a Prozac™ deficiency." Your symptoms are real—the way to recovery is contained within these pages. Someone who has been down the road of these disorders personally knows all the dark corners and has compiled her story of research and recovery, and how she incorporated it into her busy, professional life. To use the excuse, "I don't have time for all that" or "I can't afford that," is not acceptable when the quality of the rest of your life, and life itself, is at stake.

Gloria is an example of someone who lived solely on organic rice products and variations of fresh organic carrot juice, supplemented by minerals and natural remedies for months at a stretch when her body would tolerate nothing else without a violent reaction. She lost most of her hair, was thin and malnourished and generally home- and office-bound for months. Every introduction of new food was baby steps: If there's a reaction, stop! Go back! Wait a week or so and try again. Over and over this was the way she inched back into eating a more varied diet, all the while continuing her detoxification protocols. I'll never forget her excitement over having successfully consumed, with no reaction, an organic yam! Or her first scrambled organic egg! Everything that crossed her lips had to be organically grown. That meant creative solutions to the lack of local availability in a small town. Living this way took on a new meaning—no dining out, brown-bagging your lunch, dinner at someone's home, or traveling.

When compelled to make radical changes in your lifestyle and nutrition, you are actually doing your health a huge favor. These changes force you to look for, and avoid, sources of toxic substances in every aspect of your life that pervade our world today.

Gloria struggled through the food issues, and just when she thought it was safe to face the world again—wham! The fumes of traffic on the road; the smells emanating from the newer computer in her office; the mere existence of carpets and furnishing in her home; the chemical smells at the hair salon; exposure to fragrances—all began to close off more and more activities and made her examine, evaluate and modify her surroundings very carefully—as she had guided her clients to do. Computer work had to be limited to short periods; road trips were eliminated except to and from her colon and massage therapist; her hairdresser came to her home, and friends and staff did all the shopping. Does this sound familiar, is this what's happening to you?

Personally, sitting on the sidelines it was extremely illuminating as a health practitioner never exposed to clients with these disorders. Observation of her progress and recovery, through her personally designed detoxification protocols that included colon hydrotherapy, has been an eye-opening experience personally and professionally.

I had always lumped together enemas and colon hydrotherapy as in the same category as laxatives—the potential for dependency. Gloria's evolving detoxification and rejuvenation program incorporated colon hydrotherapy, an especially formulated colon fiber-cleanse tolerated by most sensitive individuals, careful nutritional and environmental modifications and specific nutrients to rebuild her health—the obvious observable health-enhancing benefits were dramatic. I soon realized, all the while she kept reminding me, of the rejuvenation benefits of reducing the overall toxic load of the body by cleansing the intestines and providing them the nutrients to detoxify and repair—she was truly an example of practicing what she teaches!

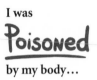
The fatigue, pain, hunger, misery, and fears experienced and shared by her have developed in me a greater empathy, sensitivity and validation for friends and those who consult with me. Her journey and anguish have already served thousands, and will, I am sure, serve thousands more. Have courage for your future, for your life. Take charge of your health and choose to be well by reading this remarkable account of a doctor who was thrust into practicing what she teaches, natural skin and body rejuvenation, and recovered.

—*Lola V. Righton, D.A.Hom.*

    Diplomate, Academy of Homeopathy

    Natural Health Consultant

2007—Gregory P. Dutson, D.C.

CAN YOU IMAGINE a life full of boundless energy, meeting each day with a spring in your step and sharp mental focus? Sometimes for people with chronic disease this may seem more like a dream than reality. Dr. Gloria Gilbère lives such a life! When she enters the room you can feel her energy. She lives a very active life, personally and professionally. The average person half her age would be lucky to keep up with her. I would have never known until I read her book that this was not always the case. Through her own dedicated medical research she developed a personal treatment and lifestyle modification protocol that not only gave her her life back, but also has the potential to help thousands of others searching to regain their health and vitality.

It is often said, "Knowledge is power." This is not accurate —applied knowledge is power. I encourage you to read Dr. Gilbère's book. Learn first-hand from her incredible journey back to health. See how she took responsibility for her own health and regained her active, vibrant lifestyle.

It is without hesitation that I encourage you to buy her book, read it, and harvest the many health related gems contained within. Isn't it time to begin your own journey back to health and vitality?

—*Gregory P. Dutson, D.C.*

Director, North Idaho Spine Clinic
Idaho Board of Chiropractic Examiners
Past Examiner and Test Committee
Member for Part IV National Board
of Chiropractic Examiners
International Continuing Education
Speaker for Health Professionals

2007—Sharon Wiseman, M.Ed.

I'VE KNOWN AND WORKED WITH GLORIA since 1990; as of the printing of this book, it's been ten years since her illness. She looks better than she's looked in years, travels around the world, and her accomplishments and bountiful energy makes her friends, family and colleagues look like we move in slow motion, compared to her. She lives what she teaches; truly an example that the age of 60 is the new 40!

—*Sharon Wiseman, M.Ed.*

Business Associate, Friend, Ergonomist,

Education Professional /Administrator 40 years

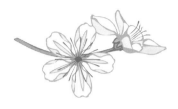

Acknowledgements

MY BUSINESS PARTNER, **Sharon Wiseman**, for her unending encouragement, support, and tireless hours spent assisting me to turn the "bitter lemons" of my medical challenges into "healing lemonade"—and make it available to all who want the recipe. Without her, my recovery and this book would not be possible.

My healing mentor, Lola Righton, who unselfishly gave of her expertise, time, energy, and friendship to open the doors to the world of homeopathy and then guided me, and pushed when necessary, to make sure I walked through.

The following people who shared their professional knowledge, time, and expertise during my illness and as part of my maintenance: Merry Alto, M.D., Marshall Arbo, D.D.S., Christopher Sturbaum, M.D., Gregory P. Dutson, D.C., and Owen Marcus, M.A., C.A.R.

My extended support group, who listened, encouraged, shared, cared and validated: Lew and Jean Mace, Tiffany Francis, Earl and Helen Heinemann, Luis and Adeline Arroyo, Christina and Ricky

Mendez, Rhonda Schnuerle, Shirley Wein, Sheri Bell-Lock, and Sharon Francis.

My organic network for providing me with healthy food, and to my delight, introducing me to new foods and preparation methods: Donna Marie McCandless, Joan Myers, Marsha Semar, Gregg Prummer, Bill and Ruth Wagner, Debbie Ackley, and the many clients and friends who shared from their respective gardens and orchards.

My publisher, Lucky Press, specifically Janice Phelps, for seeing the value of my message in publishing the first and subsequent editions of this "best selling" book.

Jan Scott—whose expertise in editing and organizing my writing for the first publication was a Godsend.

Tama Bergstrand—for her friendship and commitment to perfection, so evident in her illustrations.

Beata Golau—for fine-tuning my body during my illness, and enhancing this book with her artful illustrations.

Linda Dallmann—for her unwavering friendship and always making time to assist me with research, special projects and proof-reading.

Paz Hargrave—for being a compassionate client advocate and friend.

Bonnie Lambert—for her design excellence and insight in this new edition, and her continued support of my varied journalistic ventures.

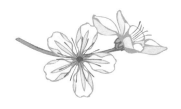

Author's Note—
Sixty *is* the New Forty

THE FOCUS OF MY WORK is education, research, and using my journalistic opportunities to spread the word about non-invasive, non-drug methods of identifying and correcting health imbalances and achieving natural rejuvenation: physical, psychological and environmental.

At this juncture of my life, the year of this publication, I celebrate **sixty years**. I am proud to have reached this milestone because my life experiences, albeit challenging, have finally become an asset rather than a liability.

Life's gained wisdom not only "set me free," it additionally allowed me to share my experiences with others. Many times my counsel provides them the light at the end of what feels like an endless dark tunnel, empty and hopeless, until someone who has walked the same path, and recovered, shines the light of validation on their dis-order, and provides them with time-tested, proven options for recovery.

Looking forward, there is so much left undone. We need to spread the word about the causes, effects and natural solutions for illnesses that destroy quality of life, yet are invisible to conventional methodologies and those not afflicted.

Together, we are the architects of the future—teaching and practicing natural health principles for ourselves, our family and future generations by additionally protecting the health of our environment, *Naturally*.

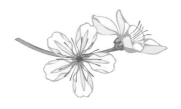

Important Note

THIS BOOK INTRODUCES ALTERNATIVE THERAPIES for leaky gut syndrome and the associated disorders. It is written to help you understand, assess, and decide appropriate treatment for a given disease or condition. The author does not intend to make comparisons between conventional and alternative medicine, other than in the context of personal experiences.

Therapies in this book are based on the training, experience, and research of the author—because each individual is so unique, the therapies may or may not be appropriate for you.

This book is not intended to replace proper medical care. Do not stop taking medications without first discussing it with a physician or health-care professional. If you decide to use any of the approaches discussed within, take this book to a physician or health-care practitioner and request referrals and cooperation in implementing natural health protocols. If a health-care professional will not, or cannot acknowledge your request, seek a health-care professional who will. It is your right to consult with a qualified health-care professional for a second or third opinion. Assume personal responsibility for your health care by becoming well-informed about available options.

Because any therapy can have risks involved, the author and publisher are not responsible for any adverse effects or consequences resulting from the use of any of the suggestions, products or procedures described in this book.

This book is not intended to diagnose, treat or cure disease, to prescribe or be a substitute for medical care. Rather, it is intended to share experiences and research and to be used as an educational tool.

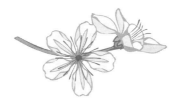

Preface (2007)

WHEN I FIRST WROTE *I was Poisoned by my body* I was director of two natural health centers that specialized in working with hypersensitive clients who didn't fit the conventional medical model. They were developing environmental and food allergies at alarming rates, and no one understood what it took to assist them to recovery—most often, not acknowledging their symptoms or that a disorder existed.

I was drafting protocols for modifications of buildings to create safe environments by using wholistic principals, and worked with general contractors and corporations to remedy sick buildings and assist their inhabitants through EcoErgonomics. My life was extremely fulfilling because I was both the building and health detective to uncover causes of health saboteurs—physically and environmentally.

After assisting hundreds of clients to wellness through detoxification, life-style and environmental modifications, clients from as far

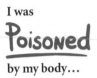

away as England, Wales, Germany, Africa, Australia, and the Middle East started to write, call and email. They consulted with me because nothing offered by conventional medicine was effective and most of them had now become allergic to medications that were offered for symptom-care by their physician.

It was challenging when I became ill and started reacting to everything. I was angry. Angry because after all the people I counseled to health, I was now having to apply those same principals to first save my life, then map out a long journey to regain my health and quality of life…this book chronicles that story.

Instead of allowing my illness to deflate my resolve, I turned my anger into positive action to live what I teach, to recover and maintain my health and…I have now done so for ten years.

After recovery and subsequently writing eight more books over the next several years, clients and readers kept calling the office asking my staff;

"How is she doing now?"

"What has she learned after all these years that isn't included in her first book?"

"Does she still use the same nutritional products as she referred to in her book?"

"What helps her clients the most for recovery?"

"Is there a common denominator in the clients that don't recover?"

"I followed her protocols and regained my life, now how do I maintain it?"

"After recovery, will I always have to be careful with products, foods, and my environment?"

"Does she still have to wear a mask while traveling? If not, what does she do to protect herself from environmental toxins and germs?"

"Does she take antibiotics? If not, what does she use when needed?"

"I heard her radio show; she sounds so energetic. How does she achieve that?"

"I heard she's been a ballroom dancer since a child. Is she able to dance after she recovered? If so, how did she build her stamina and muscle strength?"

"I knew her before her illness. She looks better now than ever. What's her secret?"

The questions referenced above are actual questions from people who communicated with my office. My intent is that all those questions, and many more, are answered in this revised, updated book.

I was compelled to write the update to *I was Poisoned* to provide a guide to wellness for the millions of people affected by chemicals of all kinds—including those our body creates internally. As I say throughout my first edition and this one as well, "Our bodies are not designed to deal with the industrialized chemicals that we bombard them with on a daily basis. Knowing how to keep your body's overall toxic load to a minimum is the only way to stay healthy in a toxic world."

In order for the first-time reader of *I was Poisoned* to follow the continuity of my health odyssey, I have left much of the original text intact. I have, however, inserted sections called "***Flash-Forward***" so that I can update information and provide progress achieved ten years later.

My prayer for you, and future generations, is that the information and experiences I share in this book will provide the motivation for you to get well and stay well, *Naturally*.

—*Gloria Gilbère, N.D.,D.A.Hom., Ph.D.*

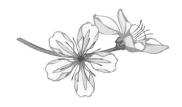

Introduction

Over the last 30 years, increasing numbers of Americans, particularly those with life-threatening illnesses, began to look for healthcare answers in complementary and alternative approaches. They are not turning their back on conventional medicine—it is, in fact, those who have had all the benefits of modern scientific medicine who have led the search—they are very much aware of its limitations and side-effects. They are exploring approaches that would complement this medicine—or in some cases, be alternatives to it.
    —Final Report of the White House Commission on Complementary and Alternative Medicine Policy, March 2002

THIS BOOK DIRECTLY CONNECTS the causes of auto-immune disorders, allergies, inflammatory diseases, multiple allergic responses, and premature aging with colon and digestive disorders. It outlines the gut causes of, and therapies for, chronic illnesses frequently mis-diagnosed or un-diagnosed. It offers safe, alternative natural choices to drug therapy.

We have become a society that expects instant results instead of taking full responsibility for our health. Doctors and health-care professionals are physicians, not magicians. The information provided here will assist you in making informed choices because after all, it's *you* who must live with the consequences of those choices. If your attitude is "give me a quick solution to get rid of my symptoms," alternative medicine is not for you—if you're "sick and tired of being sick and tired" and willing to work towards health, this book is your road map for the journey. The medical principle, "Do no harm," is honored by many of the newer concepts, based on ancient therapies, which are non-invasive. These alternative therapies have little possibility for harm and can be extremely effective.

The new paradigm in health care involves:

- active consumer involvement and responsibility for their own health
- openness on the part of patients and their physicians—abandoning narrow, restricted, "quick fix" attitudes and looking deeper for causes
- a change of attitude—honoring the ability of patients/consumers to think for themselves and know their bodies

- relinquishing the practice of disease-care that becomes symptom-care, and eventually drug-management
- a shift in belief to accept the concept of Wholistic Health—the whole person as mind-body-spirit—embracing wellness as what we eat, how we digest, utilize and eliminate it, what we believe and think, and how we move our bodies.

After reading this book, I urge you to share it with all who will listen. We are not doomed to living in a world full of chemicals that destroy our health and quality of life. There are "safe" options to toxic products. Awareness and education is the only method by which we can look forward to aging because the wisdom gained has set us free from an industrialized world that seems intent on ignoring the dangers of modern chemicals. Yes, new technologies and medications save lives and make them convenient and comfortable. However, once the world has turned against you and your immune system can no longer provide protection, you are forced to live a healthy life…if the quality of it matters to you as it does to me. Doesn't it make sense to stay healthy rather than continually struggle to get well?

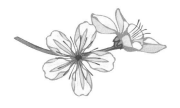

My Story

Prelude to My Story

BEING IN THE PROFESSION OF HEALTH CARE for more than 40 years, the focus of my work is education and research in non-invasive methods of identifying and correcting health imbalances: physical, psychological and environmental. As a natural health professional and recovered victim of an invisible disorder, I am proud to be living and sharing my odyssey as an example of "practicing what I teach." The following is an account of how, after a life-threatening accident, I fell into the same cycle of symptom-care as so many of my clients. It chronicles my in-depth experiences and solutions on my journey to health. This new edition shares the success of my continued wellness after ten years, *Naturally*.

My Story
Surviving on Carrot Juice and Rice is NOT Living!

Fifteen years ago I survived a life-threatening fall. As a result, I developed blood clots in my leg that became deep vein thrombosis (DVT) and eventually pulmonary embolism. After seven days in the intensive care unit, I was released...only to begin a new odyssey for which I was not prepared.

Complaints to my physician of my multiple symptoms were medically diagnosed as chronic fatigue and eventually fibromyalgia—a "catch-all" diagnosis when they didn't know what else to do. I reluctantly succumbed to prescription medications and then struggled for several months with prescription drug side-effects. The medications provided very little relief and merely served to continually bring on a new barrage of symptoms.

I eventually weaned off the medications and regained quality of life through alternative medicine and wholistic therapies. I was not prepared for what followed:

I was overdue for a long weekend respite. A colleague invited me to spend a few days in the desert. It was the middle of winter in northern Idaho—a visit to the desert was hard to resist. On the second day of my trip, I was sitting in a movie theatre when suddenly I experienced inexplicable acute pain in my right shoulder and radiating pain from the back of the right shoulder blade (thoracic area). My right hand went numb, finger mobility was lost, and the pain was intolerable. Had this been my left side, my intuition would have indicated cardiovascular involvement. My tenaciousness helped me physically get through the performance; however, my health-detective mind was preoccupied searching for probable causes. The pain continued through the evening, varying in intensity.

The next day, acute swelling manifested at the bottom of my neck. I looked and felt like the Hunchback of Notre Dame. The pain in my right shoulder blade felt like a piercing rib and as if I was walking around with a bowling ball strapped to my neck—holding up my head took enormous effort.

Four days later, I flew home and consulted with my conventional medical doctor, chiropractor, and massage therapist all without improvement or a conclusive diagnosis. Cervical and thoracic x-rays were taken to rule out any structural injury—no evident cause could be found for this debilitating pain and swelling.

After five weeks of escalating pain and impaired function, I reluctantly agreed to prescription drugs for pain management and inflammation. Shortly thereafter, I noticed my throat felt internally swollen, with no external evidence. I could swallow, but it was restricted. I mentioned these symptoms to my physician, who then suspected thyroid malfunction. A thyroid-function test showed "normal" levels. The swelling didn't escalate, but it was chronic, with few days between that were symptom-free.

Then, another symptom emerged…my hair was falling out in alarming quantities. Previously, I had enough hair for two women and very proud of it. Having witnessed this toxic drug effect in my clients, the fear of going bald escalated as my medical doctor and I kept delving for clues for an apparent cause. It is now obvious we were all searching in the wrong places.

The vicious cycle of pain, swelling, and drug side-effects continued for four months. My medical doctors were as puzzled as I. My next referral was to a neurologist to evaluate for spine involvement. The MRI showed massive swelling in the thoracic region (between the shoulders and at the base of my neck), but no apparent functional cause. My medical diagnosis was "thoracic outlet syndrome"—a fancy phrase for inflammation. At this point, while still attending to my practice, in acute pain, sleepless, and with little quality of life, *I again reluctantly agreed to prescription drug therapy*. I was prescribed a strong non-steroidal anti-inflammatory drug (NSAID). The pain was manageable with the NSAID; however, the following side-effects manifested within one week: acute constipation, abdominal cramps, bloating, accelerated fatigue, muscle pain and weakness, heartburn, "thickened throat," and heart palpitations. The symptoms were daily occurrences.

My family, friends, and clients observed the steady decline of my health. I helped hundreds of clients overcome side-effects of prescription drugs, and now I was in the same vicious cycle. Modern wonder drugs, with their toxic side-effects, took another victim, me. I spent most of my professional life searching for quality health care with safe and effective alternatives. Now I was caught up in the same web as my clients before they sought a wholistic approach to their health.

After four weeks of taking the NSAID, I started to experience rashes from foods I normally consumed. The responses manifested as profound red, hot, flushing welts in my face and neck. At times my eyes were barely visible through the swollen lids. In addition, the rashes would appear as an apparent cause of having an empty stomach. I knew these weren't female mid-life "power surges." Anxiety set in. I witnessed this reaction in my clients with food allergies—I didn't have food allergies, at least not before taking these medications. I believed I had a "cast-iron" stomach. I'd traveled all over the world; I'm a gourmet cook and love ethnic variety—eating was never a challenge. How could I suddenly be reacting to the food I'd consumed for years?

Six weeks after starting the NSAID, while eating a sandwich, my throat began to swell. I could hardly swallow. With panic in my voice, I called my medical doctor. It was conclusive I was having anaphylactic shock and needed immediate medical care—off to the emergency room I went *(flashback of symptoms reported by clients that sent them running to the hospital emergency room as well)*. Subsequently, a prescription was given for an antihistamine drug, as well as an anaphylactic injectable kit with the drug epinephrine (adrenaline)—used for generalized acute allergic reactions, especially from an insect sting. In retrospect, a drug, not an insect, had stung me. I took the prescribed medication only to have the same effects with repeated throat closures with progressive intensity and panic.

The next proposed option was a steroidal drug to control reactions. I opted to forfeit any more drugs, especially steroids. It was now painfully clear how the tangled web of prescription drugs and their side-effects catch their victims.

In addition, a new symptom developed—insomnia. This time, unlike the previous sleepless episodes caused by fibromyalgia, the insomnia was acute. This was chronic fatigue, of the mind and body, at its worst—*my mind was writing checks my body couldn't cash.*

I was afraid to eat. The same food causing an allergic response one time didn't provoke one another. I tried vegetables; some triggered a response, others didn't. Every time I attempted something new, I'd blame the reaction on that food group. There weren't a lot of foods left to experiment with and the symptoms made me more and more reluctant to try. After extensive research and consultation with professional colleagues, I initiated a diet plan to cleanse and support the body while identifying the offending foods. From past experiences with clients, I suspected leaky gut, but still didn't have confirmation. I resorted to a diet of freshly juiced organic carrots, apples, ginger, and rice. This proved to be the best tolerated and least reactive.

The malnutrition and weight loss started. Within two months I eliminated 40 pounds. All the old symptoms of fibromyalgia and chronic fatigue returned—I felt as if I was bruised all over and the nerve endings were on the surface. As if this wasn't enough, my hair continued falling out in chunks, my previously clear complexion now had acne and rashes, and my nails developed deep ridges and peeled.

Other manifestations of my malnourishment and stressed liver were the dark circles under my eyes and a yellow color to my skin and eyes. Conventional liver-function blood testing showed "within normal range." However, alternative testing showed excessive liver stress and inability to neutralize toxins.

As the condition progressed, I was more and more isolated from family and friends. I couldn't go anywhere without carrying my organic juices and rice. I had no energy to socialize. It took all my energy to continue my practice part-time, return home at the end of the day to prepare food I could tolerate, and fall into bed, though not to sleep. My nightly companions were pain, tears, and helplessness. Frustration was coupled with flashbacks of clients who shared similar stories of symptom-care. This was not living; it was surviving. Most nights I couldn't even muster enough energy for a valued telephone conversation. Friends and family kept asking, "Aren't you better yet?" So I stopped giving any details when asked, "How are you doing?" No one understood, unless they, too, had experienced an invisible illness that forced a complete life-style change.

Some people thought I went too far by refusing to eat anything non-organic. Those were the people who weren't with me in the midst of a violent reaction to non-organic foods. No, I hadn't become a health fanatic. I was struggling for survival. Previous to my illness, I took pride in maintaining my reputation as a gourmet cook, but didn't cook exclusively organic. My meals were low-fat and balanced, using organic foods from my own gardens and buying locally-grown organic produce and poultry, when available. Now, non-organic was not an option; it was essential to life. The addition of chemicals in the food, either for growing or preserving, could ultimately kill me.

Winter months in northern Idaho were the most challenging and expensive. I couldn't go to my local grocery store and buy organic foods and produce. All produce had to be special-ordered at a health-food store 45 miles away, purchased in the closest metropolitan city 125 miles away, or purchased frozen through a co-op delivery service twice a month.

Even though not familiar with many natural health protocols, my primary-care physician did everything possible within her scope of conventional medicine. I am fortunate in having a medical doctor who listens to her patients and then goes the extra mile to facilitate solutions. Many times, her solutions include referrals to alternative-medicine practitioners, even though it might go against the conventional education and consciousness of her peers. Much to her credit, when all she could offer me was more medications for symptom-care and another referral, she said, "I have no answers for you. You know more about this condition than I do."

The next suggested conventional referral was to an allergist to determine foods and substances I was allergic to. I'd been down this road with many clients who never fully recovered because the root causes were never dealt with. I was in a vicious cycle of *symptom-care, not health-care*. Disease had set in. I was again on a professional quest; this time it was for me.

So…again, I set out with the determination of a health detective to uncover clues and discover the *gut* causes of my disease.

My suspicion of leaky gut syndrome grew, but I needed to see it for myself. I scheduled an innovative blood test called a live cell analysis. I previously had this test performed on a yearly basis as a way of monitoring my health (yearly check-up).

It is accomplished through a single living drop of peripheral blood taken by a laboratory technician or practitioner from the fingertip onto a slide. It is then put under a powerful microscope, magnified up to 12,000 times and transferred to a computer monitor by way of a fiber-optic camera for easy viewing by the patient and technician. The patient is intimately involved by being able to observe immediate results (the true essence of living color)—commonly explained for education purposes by the technician and/or practitioner.

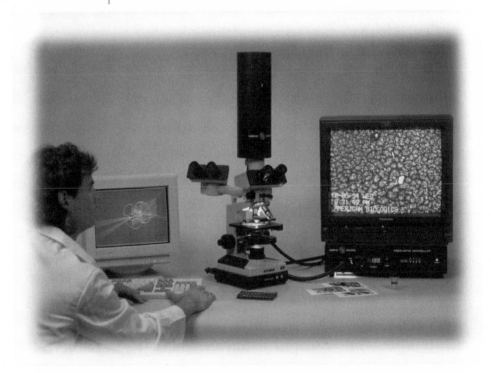

My suspicions were confirmed, leaky gut. The following photos identify the condition in the area of my intestinal tract before developing leaky gut, after developing leaky gut and the healing that occurred ten months later. This is a case where, truly, a picture is worth a million words to the patient and healthcare provider. Unfortunately, conventional medicine in the U.S. does not use this testing method, although widely used in many countries including, but not limited to, Europe, Australia, Japan and Latin America.

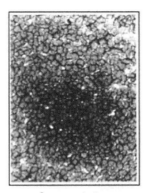

One year before
leaky gut

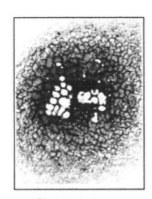

Showing leaky gut
and inflammation

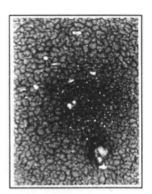

Ten months after healing
from leaky gut

Armed with photographic evidence, I now had the information that enabled me to see that my body was poisoning itself. With the revealing of this information, I started the journey of my life—to identify appropriate natural therapies providing real solutions, not band-aid drugs. I was a detective out to solve the case, my case, to heal and regain health and quality of life as I had done for my clients.

Today, ten years after this odyssey began, I've recovered—with a full head of hair, albeit grayer for the wear. Up until now, only my hairdresser knew my challenges in trying many products to find a healthy solution to cover my gray—one that was non-toxic and achieved complete coverage. I describe my preferred products later in this book. I don't mind aging, I just don't want to feel or look my age.

This publication validates those with invisible illnesses as well as clients who seek my counsel in their gut-wrenching journey to *add life to their years, not just years to their life, Naturally.*

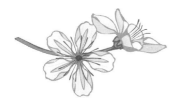

Diseases and Disorders Associated with Leaky Gut Syndrome (LGS)

LEAKY GUT SYNDROME (LGS) is a clinical disorder associated with increased intestinal permeability. Simply put, large spaces develop between cells of the gut wall. It's likened to your body's digestive filter being damaged or destroyed—allowing bacteria, proteins, toxins, and food to leak into the blood supply.

The official definition is an increase in permeability of the intestinal mucosa to luminal macromolecules, antigens and toxins associated with inflammatory degenerative and/or atrophic mucosal damage. Essentially, it represents a hyper-permeable intestinal mucosa or lining.

LGS causes inflammation of the intestinal lining and damage or alteration of the microvillus (cellular brush borders lining the intestinal tract). The damaged cells (microvillus) are then unable to produce the necessary enzymes and secretions essential to effective digestion and absorption of nutrients. This increasingly common disorder is not well known, rarely tested for, and much less understood in conventional medicine. It is estimated that over 62 million people in the U.S. alone suffer from digestive diseases, including LGS. Leakage of imperfectly digested proteins through a damaged intestinal lining is the root of many allergies and diseases. In a healthy gut, the intestinal lining is selectively porous to water and nutrients and normally resistant to most antigens and chemical toxins.

Damaged Intestinal Lining

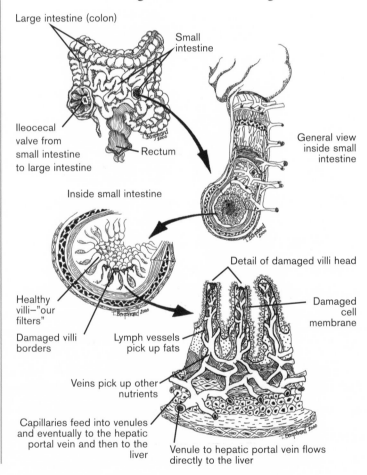

Large intestine (colon)

Small intestine

Ileocecal valve from small intestine to large intestine

Rectum

General view inside small intestine

Inside small intestine

Detail of damaged villi head

Healthy villi—"our filters"

Damaged cell membrane

Damaged villi borders

Lymph vessels pick up fats

Veins pick up other nutrients

Capillaries feed into venules and eventually to the hepatic portal vein and then to the liver

Venule to hepatic portal vein flows directly to the liver

- Anaphylactic shock
- *Candida* (yeast overgrowth)
- Celiac disease
- Chemotherapy
- Chronic fatigue syndrome
- Chronic hepatitis/ liver dysfunction
- Pancreatic dysfunction
- Colitis
- Colon cancer
- Crohn's disease
- Environmental illness/Multiple chemical sensitivities
- Fibromyalgia/Myofascial pain syndrome
- Food allergy, specific food intolerance
- *Giardia*
- Gout
- Inflammatory and infectious bowel diseases
- Inflammatory arthritis
- Irritable bowel syndrome
- Malnutrition
- Parasitic involvement
- Skin conditions: eczema, psoriasis, dermatitis, hives

Hyperpermeability (abnormal leaking) may be the primary culprit in the biological role for the evolution of each disease, or it may be a secondary consequence, causing immune system activation, hepatic (liver) dysfunction, and pancreatic insufficiency.

The leakage of toxic substances from the intestine is usually controlled by the immune system—eventually, it becomes overwhelmed. This overwhelmed system allows toxins to leak and enter the liver—

increasing overall burden, and reducing its ability to neutralize toxic substances. When the liver cannot deal with the toxic overload, it flushes it back into the blood supply, and the body's alarm systems are triggered (allergic responses).

The circulatory system, considering this as an attack to the immune system, pushes toxins to the connective tissues and muscles. This essentially is the body's attempt to store excess toxins away from vital organs to prevent major organ damage. If this condition continues, substances larger than particle size such as disease-causing bacteria, potentially toxic molecules, and undigested food particles, are allowed to pass directly through the damaged cell membranes. This, in turn, sends them directly into the blood supply—activating the alarm and causing an allergic reaction. When this alarm is sounded, the body's response is the release of histamines called cytokines. Cytokines alert the lymphocytes (white blood cells) to fight the invading particles, producing oxidants to the response and causing irritation and inflammation. These symptoms are especially evident in multiple allergic responses to chemicals, allergies, arthritis, fibromyalgia, bowel disorders, and chronic fatigue. When gut health is compromised, general health declines. *This inflammatory response is so far removed from the digestive system, the causes are usually overlooked.*

Auto-intoxication–
How the Body POISONS Itself

SIMPLY PUT, your plumbing system develops a leak, intestinal permeability, causing intestinal matter and toxins to enter circulation—rather than being properly digested and carried through the intestines (small intestine and colon) for elimination. The leaked toxins circulate to the liver, increasing its workload, and limiting its ability to neutralize toxins or filter itself efficiently. When toxins are dumped into the liver faster than its ability to neutralize them, it flushes toxins back into circulation (or stores them in soft connective tissues, manifesting as inflammation and soreness). This is done to protect vital organs—allowing time to deal with the overabundance of toxins at a later time when it's not overburdened. If toxins continue to leak through the intestinal mucosa, the liver never has the ability to detoxify what is already stored in soft connective tissues and symptoms develop as those experienced in fibromyalgia, arthritis, and lupus.

Compare this to shoving garbage down a kitchen sink, a little garbage won't hurt. At first the water still flows, although slower (the body is still operating, but with impaired function, not often recognized until specific symptoms emerge). If we continue to pack the drain with garbage, the water and waste products back up. Now we have garbage in the kitchen sink accumulating and spilling onto the floor—similar to the backup occurring within the body. When food particles are not properly digested and eliminated, they back up in the intestines and toxins leak throughout the body. Stored toxic matter causes inflammation as the body attempts to deal with these poisons—causing the eventual breakdown of the immune system.

The Role of the Large Intestine (Colon)

Trillions of cells are associated with the human body—ninety percent are bacteria micro-flora microorganisms living in the large intestine, or colon. According to the leading expert on nutrition, the late Dr. Bernard Jensen, "Bacteria in our intestinal tract weigh nearly $3^1/2$ pounds, and are metabolically active." These bacterial microorganisms are essential to life, yet it's amazing how little is known or understood by conventional health-care about their powerful role.

It is universally accepted that auto-intoxication (intestinal poisoning), with its lack of adequate health-enhancing intestinal flora, is the underlying cause of an alarmingly large percentage of degenerative disorders and symptom complexes. The colonic micro-flora is a population of its own and takes up residence within the body. We know scientifically that a balance of health-enhancing flora is imperative for health. Imbalances between the flora and the body's intestinal operating systems can result in life-threatening implications from nutritional deficiencies, allergies, infection, impaired metabolism, toxicity, and even cancer.

The Raging "Fire" Within Us— Linking Inadequate Digestion and Auto-intoxication

When the digestive system is not operating at full potential, improperly digested food molecules do not sufficiently break down for absorption across the gut wall. These improperly digested molecules are met with great enthusiasm by the "unfriendly" or "health-depleting" bacterial growth in the last section of the small intestine, the ileum. The unfriendly bacteria thrive on a banquet of food particles that are not adequately processed by the digestive system—being fed just what they need to multiply at alarming rates.

Bacteria are constant in the body—kept in balance within a healthy body by the predominance of health-enhancing bacteria. The job of these microorganisms is to create an envi-

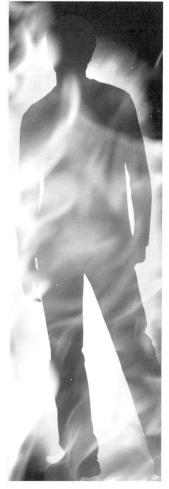

ronment that restricts growth or multiplication of health-depleting bacteria.

Lactobacilli and other forms of bacteria are the health-enhancing variety—the same bacteria that promotes souring of milk. They must be greater in number than the health-depleting variety in order for the body to digest, assimilate, and eliminate properly. When this healthy process does not occur, due to the "bad guys" outnumbering the "good guys," putrefaction occurs—the consequence of rotten food forming chemical toxins that are poisons to the body.

Metabolic "Burn-Out"

If you doubt the destruction and inflammation caused from putrefaction processes, consider this: When you stir compost waste after putrefaction, there can be sufficient heat produced by created gasses to ignite a fire. In the case of our body, the toxic material ignites a series of symptom reactions as a consequence—setting off the intestinal fire alarms in an attempt to deal with the poisons. Our internal fire manifests as symptoms—warning of impending metabolic burnout.

The chemicals produced by putrefaction are so poisonous they irritate (inflame) the delicate lining of the colon. If this condition is allowed to persist, it destroys the protective barrier keeping out the invading toxins. The damage from these toxins is so destructive the colon walls become leaky and allow penetration through the damaged barrier into the liver, lymphatic

Portal System Connecting Colon to Liver via Veins and Lymph System

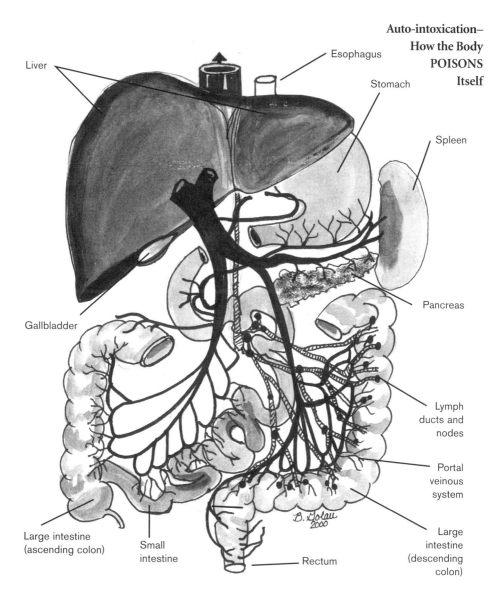

**Auto-intoxication–
How the Body
POISONS
Itself**

Liver

Esophagus

Stomach

Spleen

Pancreas

Gallbladder

Lymph
ducts and
nodes

Portal
veinous
system

Large intestine
(ascending colon)

Small
intestine

Rectum

Large
intestine
(descending
colon)

and circulatory systems. The more putrefaction, the more constipated the person. When the body becomes overwhelmed with toxins it can't handle, it becomes a raging fire on a path of self-destruction.

At this stage, the body is poisoning itself.

As the biological alarms for survival are triggered, the result is a breakdown of the immune system, resulting in numerous diseases, inflammatory disorders, food allergies, allergic reactions, and eventual death. Death may be reported to be from a specific disease, such as liver or kidney failure—not usually investigated are the initial causes leading to the disease processes.

Gut Reactions–Symptoms of Leaky Gut Syndrome (LGS)

THE FOLLOWING IS A CLASSIC LIST OF SYMPTOMS experienced with leaky gut syndrome (LGS). In most cases, LGS is the root cause often overlooked in the clinical diagnoses. Keep in mind this condition is a syndrome—stemming from multiple causes.

Symptoms of LGS

- Anaphylactic reactions
- Migraine headaches
- Acute/chronic insomnia
- Recurring skin rashes/ flushing/welts
- Sudden onset of food allergies
- Hemorrhoids
- Multiple chemical sensitivities
- Heartburn/acid reflux
- Sudden hair loss and nail changes
- Malnutrition
- Myofascial/muscle pain
- Difficulty breathing
- Abdominal pain
- Auto-immune disorders
- Mood swings/depression
- Poor exercise tolerance

- Fevers of unknown origin
- Impaired memory
- Gluten intolerance (celiac disease)
- Bloating/excessive gas
- Recurrent vaginal infections
- Swollen/sore lymph glands
- Recurrent bladder/ urinary infection
- Muscle cramps
- Excessive anxiety or aggressiveness
- Unexplained blurred vision
- Chronic fatigue
- Sleep disorders
- Liver dysfunction— pain and/or swelling/ yellow tone to skin and eyes
- Chronic constipation/ diarrhea (dependence on laxatives)
- Brain-fog—"Your mind is writing checks your body can't cash."

Auto-immune Reactions— The Birth of Allergic Responses

Allergies can be produced by an endless list of substances present in our food, water, prescription and over-the-counter medications, as well as in what we breathe, touch, and wear. Allergies are the body's reaction to antigens (foreign or unrecognized substances). When the body is in good natural health it has the ability to deal with antigens as a normal course of function. Consequently, the one symptom of inflammatory and immune disorders is the formation of antibodies in response to antigens. In LGS these materials leak across the intestinal wall and become antigens to the tissues. As the body produces antibodies to attack them, it also attacks the tissues—it is suspected this is how auto-immune diseases get their start. *The body is literally reacting to itself.* Rheumatoid arthritis, lupus, multiple sclerosis, thyroid disease, and many other debilitating conditions are fast becoming the ever-growing "incurable" diseases.

Rashes—More than Skin Deep

In my case, the rashes and blotches from LGS occurred only on the face and neck to just above my breast. However, many clients report a long history of skin disorders, including adult acne, eczema, rosacea, and psoriasis—none of which I had prior to developing LGS.

A skin disorder is the body's attempt to fight a foreign substance it is no longer capable of handling internally. In response to the invading antigen, inflammation occurs, as well as destruction of its own tissues—involving any part of the body. In LGS, the recurrent rashes are connected as much to the body's inability to eliminate toxins as to the allergic antigen itself, as in multiple allergic response syndrome (MARS).

The skin is the body's largest organ of elimination and absorption—responsible for the greatest amount of detoxification; however, most people do not consider the skin an organ.

I was

Poisoned

by my body…

Flash-Forward

After so many years of dealing with what is called multiple chemical sensitivities (MCS), a term I never felt accurately portrayed the syndromes, I coined a phrase to name these invisible disorders, "Multiple Allergic Response Syndrome," also known as MARS. The first term implies reactions to only chemical substances—not validating allergic responses that can occur to anything, even to the body itself.

In addition, the acronym describes the feelings of an individual who develops multiple reactions that defy conventional diagnosis and are not validated by loved ones and society; they feel like they're from another planet…I know, I've been to MARS and returned to earth healthier as a result of my journey.

Gastrointestinal (GI)/Digestive System 101

The core of the digestive system is the gastrointestinal (GI) tract. This tract is a long hollow tube stretching from the mouth to the rectum—beginning at the mouth where food enters the digestive system, and ending at the anus, where fecal waste is expelled. Between the mouth and anus are the esophagus, stomach, small and large intestines. The vital organs of the liver, pancreas, and gallbladder support this diverse and essential tract. Collectively, these organs make up the digestive system.

Functions of the Digestive System

As food passes through the stomach by way of the mouth and esophagus, it enters the long, coiled tube of the small intestine.

The majority of absorption takes place in the small intestine. By the action of chewing, digestive juices are secreted and food is reduced to a liquid called chyme by the time it reaches the small intestine. Digestion of carbohydrates starts in the mouth with saliva. Proteins are broken down into short-chain fatty acids (the essential ingredients of protein formation) in the stomach. Further reduction of the chyme occurs until the molecules can be properly

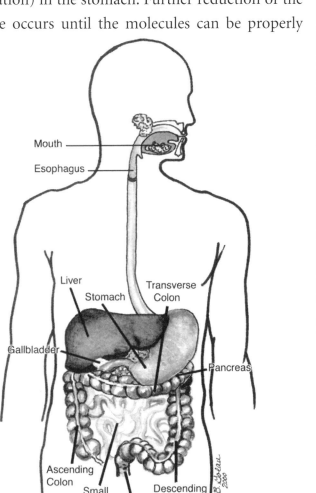

absorbed. Chyme entering through the pyloric valve from the stomach to the duodenum is highly acidic. It contains hydrochloric acid and enzymes—required to break down large molecules into smaller substances. These fluids neutralize the acidic chyme from the stomach, raising the pH from 3 to almost 8 and creating an environment better suited to lipid and carbohydrate digestion. Special cells in the intestinal wall secrete substances that combine with juices flowing from the gallbladder (bile) and the pancreas via the pancreatic duct into the duodenum.

The small intestine absorbs nutrients through the cells of the villi—acting like a strainer to protect absorption of foreign substances. **The average adult has approximately two hundred square feet of surface in the small intestine.** The small, filtered molecules pass into the cell lining (villi) and are then absorbed by tiny blood capillaries—ending up in the hepatic (liver) portal vein, where they are carried to the liver and reduced even further. This demonstrates the connection between the destruction of the villi and liver stress.

Gastrointestinal Symptoms Associated with LGS

- Abdominal extension
- Hunger pains
- Reduced appetite
- Indigestion
- Heartburn/acid reflux
- Belching/burping
- Flatulence (gas)
- Itchy anus
- Abdominal cramps/ spasms

- Anal irritation
- Alternating bowel function
- Bloating

- Constipation
- Diarrhea
- Liver pain/swelling

Constipation and Diarrhea— Essentially the Same Disorder

Symptoms of Constipation

- Painful bowel movements due to stool hardness
- Inability to execute complete elimination
- Bloating and gas
- Feeling of sluggishness

- Hemorrhoids
- Indigestion
- Depression or anxiety
- Rapid heart rate
- Tender or distended abdomen

Causes of Constipation in LGS and Related Disorders

Constipation is often induced by drugs and substances including, but not limited to, the following:

- Codeine, or other high-potency pain medications (Example: Hydrocodone APAP®)
- Antacids containing aluminum (Example: Prevacid®)
- Iron supplementation
- Drugs and substances including, but not limited to, narcotic drugs for anxiety, depression, and muscle pain (including benzodiazepines). See Resources for a complete list of benzodiazepines.

Symptoms of Diarrhea

- Frequent bowel movements consisting of watery waste matter
- Feeling like elimination is not quite complete
- Tender or distended abdomen
- Bloating and gas
- Feeling of sluggishness and fatigue
- Hemorrhoids
- Indigestion
- Depression or anxiety
- Rectal burning or itching

Causes of Diarrhea and Related Disorders

Victims of chronic diarrhea believe their colon is not constipated or impacted with toxic matter because they move their bowels several times a day. Yes, their eliminations may not be restricted or condensed, but the cause of the diarrhea is usually linked to colon irritation. The diarrhea occurs as waste accumulations adhere to colonic walls, causing irritation from accumulation of stagnant waste and the accompanying overgrowth of bacteria and parasites. As inflammation progresses, colon passageways narrow and restrict elimination of large matter, allowing only liquids to be expelled—compounding the problem of waste accumulation. Chronic diarrhea responds remarkably well to an effective fiber colon-cleansing protocol, supplemented by non-habit-forming herbal stool softeners as needed.

Food Intolerance

Exactly when an allergenic sensitivity occurs is determined by as many diverse factors as there are allergens, including duration of exposure and extent of damage. Most patients had no evidence of food sensitivities prior to LGS. However, many people report intolerance to certain foods and environmental factors after taking prescription drug medications—gut symptoms and escalating multiple responses occur later. Eating reactive foods releases irritant substances into the gut, causing inflammation. Therefore, the complex question in LGS is: Which came first, LGS or liver dysfunction?

Non-steroidal anti-inflammatory drugs (NSAIDs), while in the bloodstream and body tissues, reduce inflammation; when they reach the gastrointestinal tract they become irritants and cause damage to the intestinal lining. This, in turn, develops into a reduced capacity to deal with certain foods—the protein component of the food being the major trigger.

Flash-Back

In my case, I had no known allergies to any food or substance other than monosodium glutamate (MSG)—a flavor enhancer used is many restaurants and processed food. My MSG sensitivity manifested as migraine headaches. After taking NSAIDs and developing leaky gut syndrome, any food with preservatives or flavor enhancers caused a full-fledged anaphylactic reaction.

Gut Reactions–Symptoms of Leaky Gut Syndrome (LGS)

I was

Poisoned

by my body…

Flash-Forward

I still avoid chemical preservatives, flavor enhancers, and tenderizers, unless natural. These chemicals are toxic to even healthy individuals, albeit most don't recognize their symptoms and disorders could be related.

Being a gourmet cook, and forced to create new tasty recipes with all natural ingredients, I began my search for a natural meat tenderizer. I experimented with dozens of suggestions from fellow cooks and chefs until I finally had a "flash" one day while eating a tough steak in a restaurant.

I always take vegetable digestive enzymes with every meal. Since I consume them to assist in the "breakdown" of the food, I wondered if they would also "breakdown" the meat fiber before it was cooked. I proceeded to make a blend of olive oil, herbs of choice, lots of fresh-pressed garlic and the contents of two digestive enzymes per steak. I marinated the steak with this blend for two hours—the results were amazing! The steak was so tender in its raw stage it fell apart with probing by a fork. After grilling, the tenderness and flavor was incredible. I soon began to share this recipe with clients who were having problems digesting meat—they reported great results in ease of digestion as well as the unbelievable tenderness. My conclusion is that the digestive enzymes are actually starting the digestion process before consumption…a real treat for anyone, especially those with compromised digestion and absorption.

Any food or substance can cause an allergic reaction—excessive carbohydrate consumption and the following foods and substances are the most common:

- Artificial Sweeteners
- Corn
- Dyes/food coloring
- Eggs
- Fish
- Gluten-containing foods
- Hydrolyzed Vegetable Protein (HVP)
- Milk (and other dairy)

- Modified Food Starch
- Modified Vegetable Protein (MVP)
- Monosodium Glutamate (MSG)
- Nightshade vegetables (potatoes, tomatoes, peppers, etc. (see my website for a complete list or reference my book *Pain/ Inflammation Matters*)
- Nitrates (used in processed foods)
- Peanuts
- Pork
- Refined sugar
- Shellfish
- Sulfites (in wine and dried fruit)
- Tree nuts (pecans, walnuts)
- Soy
- Watercress
- Wheat

Multiple Allergic Response Syndrome (MARS)

I've devoted an entire chapter (Chapter 4) to multiple allergic response syndromes (MARS), a component of environmental illness (EI). In many cases, as in my own, this syndrome develops as a result of LGS, liver dysfunction, and a compromised immune system. Until gut health is addressed, eliminating environmental allergens alone will not provide a return to wellness and complete recovery.

Acute/Chronic Insomnia

Sleep disturbances are caused by such a multitude of factors it would be impossible to discuss them all in this book. The following are some of the contributing causes of sleep disturbances related to LGS and the subsequent disorders.

Causes of sleep disturbances related to LGS

- Parasites
- Dysbiosis (imbalance of intestinal flora)
- *Candida*
- Environmental and food sensitivities
- Chronic fatigue syndrome
- Auto-intoxication
- Liver dysfunction
- Fibromyalgia and myofascial pain syndrome
- NSAIDs
- Rebound effect of sleep medications (long-term use causes the condition they're meant to treat)
- Steroidal drugs, such as cortisone and prednisone

Flash-Back

I never experienced insomnia before my illness. Yes, the occasional sleepless night occurred as a result of an overactive mind or extra-ordinary stress—never lasting more than one or two nights. After my life-threatening accident, as described in Chapter 5 "How did I get this way?" and the prescription medications for pain and inflammation (including benzodiazepines "benzos"), insomnia set in. Medically, the insomnia was thrown in as part of the symptoms from the recently diagnosed fibromyalgia. The insomnia, muscle and nerve pain throughout my body became so acute I encountered weeks without sleeping more than one or two hours a night—many nights not at all.

My internist became so concerned he consulted with other specialists, while also conducting extensive personal research, only to say, "We don't know what else to do." He suggested

Flash-Back (cont.)

prescribing a stronger sleep medication and another benzodiazepine class of drug, and changing the drug when that particular formula was no longer effective—I declined. After much frustration on his part and mine, he handed me a book written by a sleep specialist, outlining several relaxation techniques. He additionally suggested enrolling in a sleep disorder clinic, for which he would write a referral. I thanked him for his extra efforts and walked out of his office determined to find real answers to my symptoms. The trigger for my leaky gut was the NSAIDs, because it was the only medication I took for an extended period of time. Additionally, after working with clients to help them overcome side-effects of benzo's, I was experiencing all the symptoms they described—I was now also a victim of damage being caused to my liver, gut and brain.

Flash-Forward

I have fortunately been able to improve the quality of my sleep by rotating several non-drug supplements such as, but not limited to, DeepDreams™ time-released melatonin tablets, Liposomal Melatonin Drops®, and Stress X ®.

I find that a complex works for about four weeks and then the rebound effect sets in and I'm awake all night again. Therefore, I advise doing as I do, rotate your sleep aids, even weekly, to avoid rebound effects. Experiment. If a complex works and then you have a sleepless night, immediately switch to another until you experience the rotation that works best for you.

Sudden Hair Loss

It's been my experience, personally and profession-ally, that certain pain and anti-inflammatory drugs are responsible for sudden hair loss. I advise anyone taking prescription medications to first identify the warnings or contraindications in the *Physician's Desk Reference* (PDR)—the "Bible" of prescription drugs, their use, and contraindications. It is available at your local library, doctor's office, bookstore, or pharmacy. The internet also has specific information sites for most drugs. If you have any questions, seek the assis-tance of your pharmacist.

Flash-Back

Sudden hair loss occurred within a short period of time after taking prescription NSAIDs. My hair was coming out in chunks. Eventually my hair had to be cut very short, and styled to "cover up" the bald areas. This is a fright-ening experience, and one that can be avoided by seeking natu-ral alternatives for pain and inflammation as described in this book and specifically in my book "Pain/Inflammation Matters."

Flash-Forward

I'm proud to report my hair grew back as thick as before my illness except for one small spot at my hair-line, for which I easily compensate. The challenge then became finding a non-toxic way to cover my now completely gray head of hair. I tried dozens of natural hair colors for over two years—nothing completely covered the gray. Finally, while on a trip to Montreal, Canada, to consult with a medical doctor friend who was poisoned by toxic mold and experiencing allergic reactions that had devastated her life and career, I realized her hair was no longer gray. I finally mustered-up enough courage to ask her what she used since she was so highly allergic to chemicals. With a gentle smile she said, "I'll take you to the natural pharmacy where I buy it and you can choose a color." She had no idea at the time what the depth of her kindness meant to the quality of my female image! The product is made in Italy but was not readily available in the U.S.—the brand I previously used was an Italian brand available in the U.S., with a similar name and box, but didn't cover my gray. I'm happy to report the product that completely covered my gray, Herbatint®, is now readily available in the U.S. at health food stores and select pharmacies. It is made with herbs in a non-peroxide, non-ammonia base with glycol as a developer. I've never had any reactions using it and neither have most of my clients.

Gut Reactions–
Symptoms
of Leaky Gut
Syndrome (LGS)

Liver Pain and Swelling— With a "Side Order" of Ribs

It is common for an LGS patient, or anyone with liver inflammation, to experience pain in the upper thoracic region between the shoulders and neck. The challenge, as in my case, was in identifying the association of the liver and ribs. As the liver attempts to deal with the toxic effects of drug therapy and resulting auto-intoxication, it can swell—placing pressure on many organs. As the following account clearly describes, the liver's diverse functions connect the digestive system to every other system in the body.

I was

Poisoned

by my body…

Flash-Back

My original symptoms of pain were all right-sided, involving my thoracic area, neck, shoulder and arm. At times, the pain was unbearable. Holding the steering wheel of my car or getting in and out of a chair was more than I could bear. No one could find an apparent cause. I kept describing my pain as if "my rib was poking through my shoulder blade from my back to my chest."

Finally, I was referred to a therapist who incorporates specialized massage techniques in her therapeutic bodywork. She is respectfully known as the "Rib Lady." The following is a synopsis of her findings during my therapy:

After an initial detailed consultation with Gloria, respectfully known by her clients as "Dr. G," I immediately suspected a misalignment of the first rib. Restrictions of the first rib are often the result of chronic contraction of the scalene muscles (Dr. G. humorously calls them scallions), which insert onto the rib. These powerful muscles gradually pull the rib up by as much as a one-quarter inch. There may be nerve irritation with local pain, as well as referred pain to the arm, neck, head, and chest. At the first session, I had her lie on the massage table—allowing better access to the rib area to confirm my suspicion, and hers, of rib-misalignment.

Since muscles move bone, I massaged the scalenes with a cross-fiber motion (a type of Myofascial Release Therapy) to reduce muscle tension—a firm, not hard, pressure is applied. Next I held the first ribs in place while she took a deep breath. The inhalation expands the rib cage, particularly the upper part, creating room for the first rib to "go home" (which it does fairly easy). On the exhalation, the rib cage contracts around the re-seated rib and aligns. Often this procedure affords instant relief, as was the case with Dr. G.

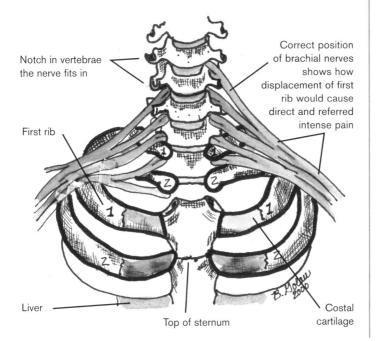

Notch in vertebrae the nerve fits in

Correct position of brachial nerves shows how displacement of first rib would cause direct and referred intense pain

First rib

Liver

Top of sternum

Costal cartilage

Gut Reactions–Symptoms of Leaky Gut Syndrome (LGS)

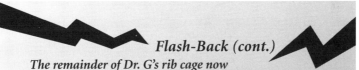

Flash-Back (cont.)

The remainder of Dr. G's rib cage now needed attention due to a right lower rib that felt like it was constantly piercing. Upon examination, there were indeed two ribs over her liver area that had moved and were pressing against one another. With a similar deep breath technique, the ribs realigned, relieving the symptom of pressure and piercing.

Continued on next page

I was

Poisoned

by my body…

In the beginning, Dr. G and I believed we found the cause of her pain, misalignment and restrictions from muscle tension. Much to our surprise, we soon learned there was a direct correlation between liver inflammation and the misalignment of her ribs. It became evident that when muscles expanded as a direct response to the inflammation of the liver, it caused contractions that resulted in the ribs being pulled out of alignment. Eventually, when her liver inflammation was under control, so was the ribs and associated pain.

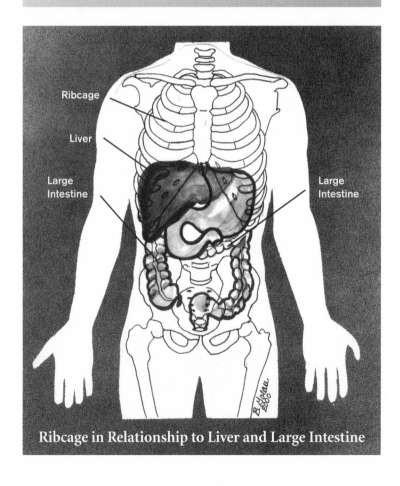

Ribcage

Liver

Large Intestine

Large Intestine

Ribcage in Relationship to Liver and Large Intestine

Flash-Back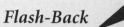

It became clearly evident that my liver involvement was a result of the prescription pain medications and NSAIDs. Most of my clients with a history of pain medications, steroidal drug therapy, or NSAIDs manifest similar symptoms, often undiagnosed by conventional methods. The majority of my clients consulted with several health-care professionals (some as many as twenty) with little, if any, improvement before seeking my counsel. It is my intent that my example will assist clients and their health-care professionals to consider these invisible symptoms with a new viewpoint—looking into functional causes rather than dispelling reported symptoms not fitting conventional diagnosis. Yes, hindsight is 20/20. Had I been able to pinpoint the cause of my initial intense pain, it would not have become necessary to take the pain medications or NSAIDs—opening the way for leaky gut and the resulting multiple allergic responses.

Flash-Forward

I still have my rib dislocate occasionally. My chiropractor applies the techniques previously described, along with his own protocols, and successfully adjusts me as needed. Now my rib doesn't dislocate as a result of liver inflammation; it occurs as a result of long hours sitting at my computer or heavy lifting (as in placing luggage in over-head storage on flights). Staying well is cost-effective and less painful than getting well. Therefore, I've incorporated chiropractic into my overall maintenance protocols. Again, the trick was finding a chiropractor that "listened" to what was previously successful, and was willing to work "out of the box" to assist me.

Brain Fog—Your Mind is Writing Checks Your Body Can't Cash

I was

Poisoned

by my body…

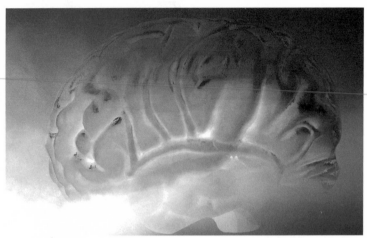

Dysbiosis (unbalanced intestinal micro-flora) is a condition resulting from the prolific enzymatic activity of the intestinal lining. In an unbalanced environment, indigenous bacteria not only make vitamins (like vitamin K) and destroy toxins, they also destroy vitamins (like vitamin B-12) and make toxins. Some by-products of bacterial activity, such as ammonia, hinder normal brain function. When absorbed into the body, the liver must remove these dangerous by-products. When the liver is not able to neutralize these substances, the results can be "foggy thinking." Brain fog, depression, attention deficit, anxiety and aggressive personality disorders are often linked to dysbiosis or systemic yeast over-growth (described in detail in Chapter 5). Brain fog can also occur as a side-effect of benzodiazepines and non-benzodiazepine sleep medications.

Anaphylactic reaction is a life-threatening condition clinically known as anaphylaxis. The word anaphylactic means it has a relationship to a substance causing the shock (reaction). The term anaphylaxis refers to a hypersensitivity resulting from contact to the reactive substance.

During anaphylactic reaction people feel anxious and can develop palpitations, tingling, itchy and flushed skin, throbbing heat in the ears, coughing, sneezing, hives, swelling, or increased difficulty breathing caused by asthma or closing off of the windpipe. Additionally, cardiovascular collapse can occur without respiratory symptoms. Usually an episode involves either respiratory or cardiovascular symptoms, not both, and the person has the same pattern of symptoms in subsequent episodes.

Anaphylactic reaction can cause a sudden drop of blood pressure and may lead to dizziness. The reaction may progress so rapidly it leads to collapse, convulsions, loss of bladder control, unconsciousness, or stroke within one to two minutes. Anaphylaxis may prove fatal unless immediate emergency treatment is given. (*The Merck Manual of Medical Information*, 1997).

In LGS, the causes of anaphylactic reactions become complicated. A response to a specific food is blamed solely on the food—seldom linked to a medication or environmental exposure, hours or days earlier. In my case, anti-inflammatory medications caused LGS which overburdened the liver, the LGS caused food allergies and the subsequent multiple allergic responses.

I was

Poisoned

by my body…

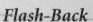

Flash-Back

My first experience with throat-closure appeared after taking NSAIDs. Subsequently, anaphylactic reaction resulted after eating specific foods, as well as from having an empty stomach—my body began reacting to itself. In addition, as my liver became over-worked and less able to process toxins, I began to experience anaphylaxis when exposed to any man-made chemicals. I was forced to eliminate everything possible in my home and office that wasn't natural and fragrance-free.

Flash-Forward

I have only experienced anaphylactic reactions a handful of times since my recovery—triggered by an unsuspecting pesticide exposure or additives in restaurant food. I still never leave home without my homeopathic complex for allergic responses as my natural "crutch." I can detect environmental chemicals a mile away, allowing me to avoid putting myself in harm's way.

One pesticide exposure was a result of a neighbor using it around his garden without warning me, as has been requested on numerous occasions. I have since moved into a planned development where restrictions are strictly adhered to.

During a trip to Florida for a conference, I unknowingly walked out of the hotel and encountered the tanker truck spraying for mosquitoes. My face turned beet red and welts emerged. I immediately returned to my room, took my high potency vitamin C powder and the homeopathic complex for allergic reactions, and the symptoms disappeared before escalating into anaphylaxis.

Not all people with digestive disorders and LGS develop severe allergic responses, however, many do.

Individuals with food allergies may react violently to eating even tiny amounts of the offending food. As an example, stirring a food that triggers an allergic response, then using the same utensil to stir or serve a tolerated food, can cause an allergic response. The small amount of offending food remaining on the utensil may never be suspected as a response trigger. To further complicate the syndrome, many people react to certain foods because the weakened digestive system lacks an enzyme necessary for digesting that specific food group.

Food additives are a huge contributor to adverse allergic responses and anaphylaxis. Major contributors to food reactions are monosodium glutamate (MSG), food preservatives such as sulfites, artificial sweeteners and dyes. Chemicals and fragrances found in many products such as candles, soft drinks, and clothing, to mention a few, add to the complex reactions associated with MARS.

Heartburn/Acid Reflux

The glands of the stomach produce a multitude of substances, including hydrochloric acid and various food-digesting enzymes.

Heartburn (also called "acid stomach") is a burning pain that spreads across the chest as acid backs up into the esophagus. It is defined as gastroesophageal reflux disease (GERD) when the stomach's contents back up into the esophagus. Symptoms generally occur after a meal and especially when lying down—which is why most symptoms are experienced at bedtime. Food allergies, improper chewing, a toxic colon, and lack of digestive enzymes are contributing factors. Once the acid has irritated the delicate lining of the esophagus and stomach, the inflammation must be halted to avoid further potentially serious problems (see *Fast-Forward* for my solution).

A faulty digestive and elimination system allows fermentation of food in the stomach and colon. Fermentation in the colon produces hydrogen methane and carbon dioxide that feed bacteria, create gas, bloating, and eventually LGS. This overgrowth of "unfriendly" intestinal flora then becomes known as dysbiosis.

Antacids, including drugs such as Prevacid®, Tagamet®, and Zantac®, are some of the common conventional treatments for heartburn/acid reflux. These medications are generally effective based on the theory that the pain of indigestion and heartburn is due to excess stomach acid. Clinical studies conducted in 1990 showed antacids were of **no real benefit** for the majority of patients with heartburn—they may provide some immediate relief, however, do not address the underlying causes. Granted, the use of antacids increases the production of hydrochloric acid by the parietal cells breaking down food for digestion. However, the cells producing hydrochloric acid become so overworked they produce less and less hydrochloric acid, creating a rebound effect.

Another side-effect of antacids is their ability to decrease protein-digesting enzymes, such as protease, already deficient in digestive disorders. Antacids are alkaloid buffers that neutralize acids and raise pH. Proteases, such as pepsin, require low

Flash-Forward

I tried every natural solution I knew of to reduce the symptoms of heartburn as well as repair damage from internal inflammation. I used different varieties of aloe juice, knowing that for centuries it has been effectively used both for internal and external healing from irritation and burns. Every brand I tried produced some type of allergic response—my clients reported the same experiences.

Finally, I located an aloe juice that is supplied only to health-care professionals and is fractionally distilled from aloe vera leaves. It is completely free of any taste, preservatives, coloring or additives. It looks, feels, and tastes like water and requires no refrigeration. It's called "Professional's Care" and not sold over the counter. I carry a small bottle whenever traveling, for those instances food I haven't prepared causes irritation or GI distress.

I find that taking two ounces (a shot glass works great), before each meal and at bedtime, provides relief and facilitates healing. My clients and readers buy it in quarts and are amazed at its effectiveness. After extensive research, I now believe it's the preservatives and coloring in other products and the potential microscopic bacteria that form which my clients and I react to—not the aloe vera juice itself. Clients with ulcers, irritable bowel, celiac disease, Crohn's disease and GERD report substantial, if not complete, relief after taking it regularly for approximately ninety days (see Resources).

pH environments for effectiveness. The antacid does not destroy the enzyme; it destroys the environment for effectiveness—for example, freezing does not destroy water, it reduces its ability to flow.

Dehydration/Mineral Loss

Intestinal disorders, particularly LGS, generally create a mineral deficiency.

See "Supplementing Minerals My Whey" in Chapter 7 for details on mineral/electrolyte supplementation.

Flash-Back

At the onset of my leaky gut, I had severe muscle cramps, commonly known as "charley horses," in the calves of my legs. There were many nights I sat in bed screaming with intolerable cramps, muscle pain and coldness in my legs—it felt as if I had an I.V. of ice water running through my veins. A patient with fibromyalgia, leaky gut, or withdrawal from benzo medications understands the type of pain I'm describing. The pain is deep-seated within the muscles and generally chronic late in the day, when weather changes, and at night. It's a feeling of "hurting and soreness all over" with no visible evidence! Once I started mineral replacement, yesterday's symptoms became today's learning experience to share with my clients and anyone who would listen.

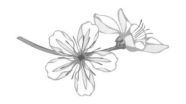

Multiple Allergic Response Syndrome (MARS)

AS IF HAVING LEAKY GUT SYNDROME (LGS) and the resulting food allergies isn't enough, multiple allergic responses to environmental factors, also known as environmental illness (EI), usually develop as well. MARS is marked by *multiple symptoms* in *multiple organ systems* (usually the neurological, immune, respiratory, skin, gastrointestinal, and musculoskeletal). MARS is a side-effect of a weakened immune system that is not able to neutralize toxins in a chemical world.

MARS is an adverse reaction to toxic chemicals in air, food, medications, supplements, fibers or water at concentrations generally considered harmless to the healthy population. However, when a healthy body is repeatedly exposed to toxic chemicals, the body develops a decreased tolerance—leading to auto-immune disorders. The more a compromised immune system is exposed to chemical substances, *the sicker the body becomes*, and may even die from the resulting allergic responses.

People with MARS manifest acute sensitivity from natural gas fumes, gasoline, car exhaust, dyes and chemicals in fabrics, clothes and fabrics containing synthetics, carpets, cleaning materials, phenolated compounds, perfumes and fragrances, smoke from cigarettes or other sources, paints/stains and construction materials, to mention a few.

21st Century Human Canaries

After World War II, a new generation of chemicals were synthesized, including pesticides, synthetic fragrances, cleaning products, food preservatives/flavor enhancers/coloring, and detergents—many petrochemicals (petroleum based) and very toxic to humans. I call them "baby boomer bombs." Theron G. Randolph, M.D., then a professor at Northwestern University, first described EI in the 1950s, when it was considered the Twentieth Century Disease. These chemicals were, and still are, considered "safe, until proven toxic." As a side-effect of our modern industrialized society, we are all participants in a global chemical experiment, and it's making millions of us, and our planet, very sick.

In the past, coal miners didn't need high tech equipment to measure air quality—they simply took a caged canary with them into the mine; if the bird stopped singing or died, the air was toxic and they got out. People with MARS are the human canaries of the 21st century, warning that the air in our homes, offices and environment is toxic. If those of us with MARS continue to be exposed to toxic chemicals, we can become dead canaries, rather than the wounded canary serving as early-warning systems through our allergic responses.

According to studies conducted by the California Department of Health in 1995 and published in *Multiple Chemical Sensitivity Research Reports,* 17%-34% of Americans report symptoms of chemical sensitivity. The studies also show that two-thirds of patients with MARS have been diagnosed with chronic fatigue syndrome and fibromyalgia. Furthermore, it is estimated that 50% of office visits in general practice today are related to complaints of food and environmental allergies.

As the gut heals, and we minimize or eliminate exposure to toxic substances, support the body's detoxification, digestion, assimilation and elimination, the symptoms of fibromyalgia, chronic fatigue and MARS are dramatically reduced and often eliminated—I'm a prime example. Reduction of toxic exposure facilitates healing by reducing the body's total toxic load. After my recovery, and counseling thousands of clients to wellness, the dramatic improvement of secondary symptoms adds support to my methodology that demonstrates these syndromes have a "gut cause."

Intolerance vs. Allergic Response

Allergies occur at any stage in life and include essentially all disorders of the immune system that involve a heightened sensitivity to substances. The distinction between being allergic to something and having a poor tolerance is extremely important—in either case, you *must* avoid the substance. Especially in LGS and MARS, as with any disease that compromise the immune system, the continued total accumulated exposure (TAE) may turn from intolerance to a life-threatening response. For example, if you're intolerant of penicillin, the symptoms may be diarrhea—if you're allergic to it, the reaction may kill you. Today, it is estimated that over 1500 deaths occur every year from penicillin reactions that lead to anaphylaxis, and that accounts for just one substance.

Symptoms of MARS

The symptoms of MARS generally start slowly. At first you may notice an increased sensitivity to environmental smoke or fragrances. It starts out simply—being extra sensitive while walking by a perfume counter, candle department, or a recently cleaned or remodeled room. Initial symptoms may include a headache, itchy eyes or skin. As the body's toxic load increases, exhaust from cars may now precipitate a rash, shortness of breath, or the immediate need for fresh air. Chemicals such as hair spray, hair color, permanent waves, deodorant, nail products, glass and bathroom cleaner, or nonstick cooking spray all produce some type of allergic response. Pesticides used on a lawn may trigger a reaction and, at first, may be brushed off as hay fever or seasonal allergies. Most people with MARS manifest escalating intolerance to loud noises, bright lights, and extremes of heat and cold. It *appears* that we suddenly react to a variety of inhalants, chemicals and mold, not identified before developing LGS.

There are two main types of allergic/hypersensitive responses.

Type One Allergic Response

Type one is an immediate-onset allergy. This is the mechanism that binds immunoglobulin E (IgE) antibodies to a specific antigen (a food or inhalant). When white blood cells are sensitized to produce the specific IgE antibodies and then contact the specific antigen, the cells in defense release powerful substances. When produced in excess, these substances are destructive and inflammatory, produce symptoms usually within thirty minutes, and damage normal tissues. These substances include lysosomal enzymes, histamine, toxic oxygen radicals, arachidonic acid, leukotriences, kinin, and bradykinin-like substances, as well as dehydroascorbic acid. The lysosomal enzymes literally digest and destroy tissue. Histamine causes leakage from capillaries, producing swelling, constriction of bronchioles, excessive mucus production, and much more.

Environmental allergens can be anything you breathe or touch, such as pollen, perfume, chemicals, or smoke. The following is a limited list of symptoms resulting from the excessive release of inflammatory substances after exposure.

Responses to Environmental Allergens

- Accelerated response to heat
- Anaphylactic shock
- Anxiety or panic attacks
- Asthma attack
- Chills
- Difficulty breathing or immediate need for fresh air
- Edema (swelling)
- Heart irregularities
- Hives/rashes
- Intestinal spasms
- Itchy eyes
- Memory loss/brain fog
- Mood swings (depression, extreme highs and lows)
- Muscle aches or cramping
- Nasal discharge/ post-nasal drip
- Sensitivity to weather changes
- Sinus congestion
- Sudden acute headache
- Tingling or numbness on tongue, face or lips

These reactions are considered non-IgE reactions and therefore are not a true allergy, but produce an allergy-like response. These reactions involve IgG antibodies, IgG immune complexes, IgM and IgA antibodies, and cellular T-lymphocyte mediated responses. These responses all have delayed onset of symptoms, usually 48-72 hours or more, after eating the allergic food or exposure to airborne allergen— most difficult to specifically diagnose.

These responses are as destructive as Type One, possibly more significant, because of the masked underlying culprit contributing to serious chronic and auto-immune diseases. The next time you feel spacey, dopey, extra anxious, or unable to concentrate, retrace the exposures of the previous few days. For many people with LGS, fibromyalgia, chronic fatigue and MARS, the delayed symptoms accelerate the generalized muscle pain and fatigue, making it harder to identify the culprit. If conventional drugs are prescribed to treat symptoms the sick get sicker. If you suspect delayed onset of symptoms, consider the following:

Were you:

- In a room with new carpet or rugs?
- In a new or recently remodeled building?
- Exposed to a new computer, copier or electronic equipment?
- Exposed to new paint or varnishes?

Multiple Allergic Response Syndrome (MARS)

- On a recently fertilized lawn or golf course?
- In a hardware, automotive, or paint store?
- Recently in a dry cleaning establishment?
- In a barber or beauty salon?

Do you:

- Have new furniture (wood or upholstered)?
- Have new draperies or synthetic window coverings?
- Microwave food in plastic containers, especially styrofoam?
- Have a new electric or gas stove?

Did you:

- Visit a hospital or medical building?
- Purchase a new synthetic pillow, mattress pad, blanket or mattress?
- Polish your shoes indoors?
- Spend time in a moldy basement or building?
- Have recent exposure to a wood-burning stove or fireplace?
- Recently use a self-cleaning oven?

Have you:

- Visited a fabric department or fabric store?
- Slept on new bedding (not washed before use)?
- Recently cleaned the interior of your car?
- Recently purchased a new vehicle?

My intent in relating this information connecting MARS and LGS is to promote awareness of the myriad causes of allergic responses. My goal is to help you take control of your life, heal your immune system, and again enjoy quality of life.

Effects of MARS

The damage to the detoxification system, especially the liver and lymphatics, may eventually extend to all body systems because they are inter-dependent. If the liver is unable to detoxify (break down) and use a chemical, the chemical ends up floating around the circulatory system, available to every cell. If damage occurs in the musculoskeletal system, symptoms may result in chronic pain and weakness, as experienced in fibromyalgia and chronic fatigue. If damage occurs in the nervous system, symptoms may include depression, anxiety, brain fog, and feeling "spacey." If the damage is in the respiratory system, the symptoms may propel a sudden onset of acute asthma or chronic bronchitis.

Life with MARS—Life-Altering

A combination of food and environmental responses alters a life like no one can imagine, unless actually experienced. Any environment beyond our control becomes a huge risk until the immune system detoxifies and repairs. A stroll in a shopping mall or store is no longer predictable. You may have to resort to e-shopping or catalog buying for awhile (assuming you don't react to the ink). Even a routine haircut has added consequences, maybe even life-threatening.

I was

Poisoned

by my body…

Flash-Back

Within minutes of entering the beauty salon, I became so hypersensitive that my face itched, turned red and I developed a terrible headache. At first, I tried to "tough it out." Eventually, a visit to the beauty shop heightened my sensitivity to other substances for days. It wasn't worth it! Being sensitive to my challenge, my hairdresser scheduled my appointments first thing Monday morning. This schedule allowed the salon to "air" a bit, after being closed on Sunday, and before the daily buildup of hair spray, perm solutions, hair color, nail products, and the multitude of chemicals associated with the beauty industry. This scheduling was effective for a while, until I became so sensitive I resorted to having my hairdresser make home visits. This much appreciated arrangement allowed me to minimize my exposure until my health improved.

Flash-Forward

My hairdresser now covers my full head of gray hair with an all natural permanent hair color made in Italy by Herbatint®. They have a variety of 30 shades and my hair is healthier and shiner than ever. As mentioned elsewhere in this book, be aware of similar names also made in Italy, with even a similar color packaging…they are NOT the same.

I go to the beauty salon regularly. However, I had to make sure the salon did not offer acrylic nails because those chemicals still induce an allergic response, although not anaphylaxis.

I only use chemical-free hair products, organic ones when possible—readily available at natural markets and pharmacies. I use toluene- and formaldehyde-free nail enamel and polish remover with no negative responses.

People facing these daily challenges get very discouraged—a new set of symptoms emerges weekly, daily, and even hourly until the allergens are identified and avoided, the overall intestinal toxic load is reduced, and the body repairs.

Stress—Adding Fuel to the Fire

Seemingly unrelated exposures and events trigger symptoms. Prior to developing LGS, a stressful situation might have been just that, a situation. Now the added component of toxic overload (intestinal and environmental) can cause a myriad of symptoms, including rashes and swelling of the throat. This response occurs because stress releases toxins and

Flash-Back

I encountered inter-personal situations that became so challenging during my illness, I had to completely discontinue communication with the individuals. The situation is especially difficult when it involves family members. We need people we care about to understand or at least be emotionally supportive; it's heartbreaking when they are not.

To the individuals pushing my "stress" buttons, my decision to eliminate stressful situations by refusing to engage in further confrontations appeared to be "selfish" and "self-serving." It was! Selfish, because I chose to take whatever measures were necessary for survival. Yes, self-serving, because I was determined to conquer this depilating disorder, help others as a result of my experience, and take back control of my life and health.

I was

Poisoned

by my body...

Flash-Forward

It wasn't until I became ill that I realized the real lack of information and ignorance about what I call invisible illnesses caused from exceeding the body's capacity to neutralize and eliminate its toxic load. Clients relayed stories of how their spouses, children, family, friends, co-workers and employers were not supportive during their allergic responses—most times believing they were complaining about a set of symptoms that was imagined or created to attract attention. I'm here to tell you, these disorders are real! I encourage you to never judge another until you've been in their same situation.

Today, I enjoy life, support the efforts of my clients to repair their health and life, validate their challenges, and *very selectively* choose my business associates, friends, people I create interpersonal relationships with, and family members I stay in touch with. If someone is not supportive—I smoothly slide out of their life and seek those that are. I live my life by reminding myself that "I can afford anything in life, except being around negative people."Negativity is a contagious disorder that is totally preventable by avoidance!

the body systems are already overloaded in dealing with LGS, a compromised liver, and the resulting disorders.

The connection between the mind and the immune system is an important one. This does not mean the immune system's reaction is "psychological." In allergic responses to emotional stress, the immune system responds by activating protective mechanisms (responses) to warn of impending danger.

According to Dr. Hans Selye, pioneer in studies of the physical effects of stress, the initial changes taking place in response to stress (a surge of adrenaline, increased heart rate, rash) are designed to help you escape a dangerous situation. The situation may be social, such as anger or fear, or physical such as nearly escaping or being a participant in an accident. Fear and anger act on the autonomic nervous system, controlling the functions of internal organs, blood components, and lymph vessels. In severe cases, emotional stress can bring on anaphylaxis, the systemic allergic reaction where airways swell and close; the person may even go into shock or die. The overall effect of stress cannot be taken lightly.

Different Day, Different Symptom

Because individuals are so biochemically different, there are tremendous variations in responses to chemicals—the environment is always changing, so are the responses. Substances may cause a reaction one day and not another. Total accumulated exposure (TAE) creates a decreased tolerance. Therefore, the more we're exposed, the less we tolerate.

No two people encounter the same reaction to environmental conditions. MARS and EI can be difficult to diagnose because of varied symptoms. Routine blood tests frequently indicate no problem exists. Fortunately, there are more and more medical and health-care professionals who do recognize these disorders usually have a gut cause. Many clients are treated with drugs for digestive disorders, only to be given more drugs when multiple allergic responses develop—emphasizing symptom-care rather than health-care. Yes, drugs save lives (including my own). That said, it is my opinion they should be used for acute care, not symptom-care that becomes drug-management—and then only until root causes are identified and natural solutions initiated.

The key to wellness lies in minimizing and reversing damage to body systems by avoiding or limiting continued exposure to toxic elements. In today's toxic environment everybody appears fated to suffer some form of MARS or EI. The only way to effect positive changes is through education and personal responsibility. Each person's total accumulated exposure (TAE) is like a volcano—building excessive gasses in the gastrointestinal tract, waiting until the pressure must be released to erupt with an allergic response. At first exposure, we may develop minor allergies. Eventually, the immune system is so over-worked the allergies become acute.

Your Internal Toxic Tocsin (ITT)

When people become sensitized to chemicals, they react at levels not detectable by others. I refer to this as the "internal toxic tocsin (ITT)." A tocsin, according to Webster's, is an "alarm or signal." The word originated from the Spanish *tocar*—meaning to touch or ring a bell. Just as a smoke detector is triggered by smoke as a warning of impending danger, your ITT is the body's alarm system signaling toxic overload, as experienced in allergic responses.

Life is no longer ordinary, even though on the outside we may *appear* just fine (unless you're like I was, yellow with jaundice, swollen with rashes, and suddenly 50 pounds lighter). When someone has a visible challenge (broken limb or paralysis), the seriousness leaves little to question or doubt. When we're challenged with multiple syndromes (LGS, fibromyalgia, chronic fatigue, MARS and EI) the effects are not immediately evident to the observer, and if they are, they occur during the allergic response and then visibly disappear. In some, the resulting skin disorders are always present in varying degrees. At the first sign of an allergic response, the victim *must* alert others that internal swelling and restricted breathing is occurring (unless they're unable to speak while gasping for air and grabbing their throat). If you ever witness someone in the midst of an anaphylactic reaction, it's a terrifying experience you won't soon forget!

Your ITT may also respond by producing excessive mucus, nasal congestion, bronchial constriction,

Multiple Allergic Response Syndrome (MARS)

Internal Toxic Toscin (ITT)

I was

Poisoned

by my body...

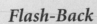

Flash-Back

For several months, my housemate and I detected strong chemical odors penetrating the house late at night. It was an inconvenience; however, the implications of long-term effects were not immediately evident.

It is not unusual in a rural farm area to experience heavy smoke from field and slash burning, so we dismissed it as a seasonal nuisance that would eventually go away.

At first, our symptoms were minor, a slight headache and sore throat. Then, as exposures continued, every time the smell was detected we developed a headache, nasal congestion, and excessive mucous (indicating decreased tolerance).

Shortly after my diagnosis of leaky gut, I experienced my first frightening reaction to environmental exposure. Since developing LGS, I had first-hand experience with anaphylactic reactions from foods not tolerated, but not from environmental allergens. One night I was awakened by an especially strong toxic odor penetrating the open window in my bedroom. Within 10 minutes, my face began to swell and itch, I developed a pounding frontal headache, and my throat swelled. I knew something extremely toxic was burning; the smell was the same as in the past, only now much stronger. I was again forced to be a health detective...the investigation started. The only clues: a neighbor still burned his trash, the smell was always late at night, and the odor was stronger on cloudy nights. That evening, after assisting me through the anaphylactic reaction, my housemate followed the toxic smell outdoors. Indeed, a neighbor was burning trash. To make matters worse, deeper investigation uncovered evidence of burned plastics and automobile oil filters. The individual acknowledged responsibility and stopped burning. However, the exposure triggered serious allergic responses to environmental allergens not previously experienced. My already toxic body had reached its maximum capacity to neutralize chemicals from the exposure.

This neighbor was not only putting our health at risk, he was polluting the environment and possibly other individuals who experienced allergic responses without tracing it to a toxic airborne substance in their neighborhood.

103

Multiple
Allergic
Response
Syndrome
(MARS)

itching, or headache. These alarms, although not immediately as serious, are still warnings.

For me, as for the millions with these disorders, drastic measures must be taken to control toxic exposure, nutritionally and environmentally. These measures are essential to survival, function, and restoration of health.

A client relayed another case of potentially life-threatening toxic exposure caused by an individual insensitive to implications of their actions:

During a commercial flight, a woman passenger was removing her nail polish. Many nail-polish removers and nail polishes contain toluene, a known carcinogen, as well as other toxic chemicals like acetone. The use of this substance in an enclosed airplane cabin with re-circulating air makes this situation extremely dangerous. The woman passenger was annoyed when asked, by my client, to refrain from using the substance because of its toxic nature and the risk posed to passengers and crew, especially those with heightened sensitivities. This seemingly innocent act had the potential for devastating consequences.

It is alarming to imagine the unsuspecting pollutants inhaled from an airborne toxin during a routine airplane flight. What should be of equal concern is that this type of hazard *can* be completely avoided, if people take responsibility for the substances they use and the potential hazards posed to people and

I was

Poisoned

by my body...

Flash-Forward

As soon as I regained my health, I moved from the rural community to a city 35 miles south. To avoid dampness and mold, I found a custom-built 20-year-old home with no basement, in a private community nestled in evergreens with fresh air by the lake and... with strict regulations. I interviewed several contractors before deciding who was best suited to take on my project. The contractor I chose was willing to work with my requirements in spite of not having in-depth knowledge of the needs of highly sensitive individuals or of non-toxic building materials and protocols.

Fortunately, as an eco-environmental consultant and real estate investor, I've been involved in building or remodeling over forty structures within the past forty years. I was knowledgeable about what had to be done and what was needed for it to be "safe." Much to the credit of my contractor and newfound friend, Skip Pucci, he took extra measures to protect my health, and admitted what a learning experience my project became. After more than thirty-five years in the building industry, he now has first-hand experience and sensitivity to the needs of MARS and EI victims and uses it to build healthier homes and offices in the greater Sandpoint area of Idaho.

It took me six long months with a full crew to have the house renovated, down to bare 2 x 6's, all with non-toxic materials. I allowed the house to off-gas for a couple of months while maintaining a high indoor temperature to help "cure" everything new before moving in.

I love my new home, its location, and community—a testament to my recovery. In order to maintain my health and still do all the travel my profession requires, I live by the 80/20 rule: 80% of the time I live a healthy, organic, non-toxic life— the other 20% I have limited control. This ratio protects against exceeding the body's ability to protect me, and a healthy rule for you to live by after your recovery.

105

Multiple
Allergic
Response
Syndrome
(MARS)

the environment. As more and more people respond to environmental pollutants, education is the master key to prevention. Knowledge is power, power to protect and heal ourselves and the environment. The power to eliminate toxic pollutants begins when consumers refuse to buy or use products that are not natural. In this way we *do* make a difference, one person at a time.

After relating the above story to another client, she described a specific incident experienced with nail polish remover, confirming its level of toxicity. She was using polish remover in her bathroom, and it activated the carbon monoxide detector. The incident initially peaked her concern then soon forgotten until we entered into a discussion about my increasing sensitivities to commonly used highly toxic chemicals. Our conversation stirred my insatiable curiosity. So, I again became the health detective and asked a science teacher to conduct the same test with another brand of nail-polish remover—the toxic ingredients again triggered the detector.

Toluene is a liquid hydrocarbon (C_7H_8), resembles benzene, is flammable, is a toxic solvent, and used as an anti-knock additive in gasoline. Hydrocarbon is a constituent present in petroleum, natural gas, and coal. I rest my case for the seriousness of generalized toxic exposure to chemicals like toluene, especially in a public area in an enclosed space with re-circulating air. I hope this example will raise individual awareness and responsibility to the potential risks posed by substances that we routinely use.

The following account chronicles my personal experience with toxic re-circulating air.

Flash-Back

I was scheduled for a routine dental cleaning in an office I had visited many times the past several years. On this particular visit, and after developing LGS and MARS, I entered the reception area, announced my arrival, and proceeded to read a magazine while waiting to be called for my appointment.

Within a few minutes, my face was itching, it turned red, and I developed a stabbing frontal headache. When I relayed my symptoms to the hygienist, she commented that she and several staff members were recently experiencing symptoms of headaches and red, irritated eyes. There was no new equipment or dental products in the office. She suspected something toxic was circulating from within the medical building where the dental office was located. We decided to proceed with the dental cleaning, since I had traveled two hours, and it would be months before I could be rescheduled. The hygienist was not finished when I exclaimed, "I have to get out of here." By the time I left, my eyes looked as if they were painted red, my throat felt as if it was sandpapered, and a rash was progressing down my neck as the headache continued to pound.

After leaving the building, I took my usual homeopathic remedy for allergic responses and walked in the fresh winter air. Soon acute symptoms subsided. While eye redness disappeared within a couple of hours, the headache and sore throat continued. Within three days, I had lumps the size of golf balls in my throat; my lymph system was swollen from

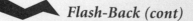

dealing with the extraordinary load of toxins.
The lingering effects from the exposure in the dental office building continued for three weeks, along with a sore throat, muscle pain and fatigue. I was a "lucky canary;" I fled the building, just in the knick of time.

There was definitely something very toxic circulating within that building. The office is located in a large multi-use medical facility and the ventilation system is interconnected. The exact source of the pollutant is difficult to detect. My experience added validity to the concerns and symptoms of the employees and prompted a search for the toxic origin. I became the internal toxic tocsin, early warning of danger lingering in the air. In this instance, I became the "wounded canary"—fortunately not a dead one.

Weeks later I had occasion to speak with the hygienist. She confirmed that upon investigation the cancer center in the building was using some new kind of chemical and it was apparently circulating throughout the professional building. Because of the complaints of multiple symptoms from the occupants of the building, the cancer center was asked to provide a filtration system to their facility. I have no idea if anyone truly resolved the issue; however, rest assured, I never returned to that building.

Digging Your Teeth Into
Multiple Allergic Responses

During the 1960s and 70s I worked in dentistry. I had all the amalgam (silver) fillings and other restorations removed and replaced by gold, composite, or a combination of alloy and porcelain. No one suspected that years later the alloys used in dental restorations would be detrimental to health. In individuals with weakened immune systems, like LGS, MARS and EI, the reaction to alloys can cause an array of reactions, some serious.

After developing LGS, I developed gingivitis, an inflammation of the gums. This was not surprising, because oral health is one of the first indicators of a weakened immune system and poor nutrition. The gums were so sensitive it was torture to brush, much less use toothpaste. I finally resorted to baking soda and salt, which still caused discomfort, but to a lesser degree.

Attempts by my dentist, hygienist, and me to eliminate the inflammation were unsuccessful. Finally, when my LGS improved substantially, so did the inflammation. However, two teeth remained chronically inflamed. The surrounding tissues were bright red, swollen, and bled from the slightest pressure.

The two teeth involved were my upper cuspids (eye teeth). They were restored in 1966 using porcelain fused to metal. The metal used was an alloy base containing titanium; the porcelain was baked over the crown cast of metal. At the time of restoration, this type of porcelain crown was the best. Since I worked in the office that prepared and made the crowns, I discussed my restorative options with the dentist and lab technician. I decided on titanium, since it was the dental metal of choice for restorative dentistry in the 60s. I recall joking about the potential of titanium setting off metal detectors—little did I know what physical alarms it would trigger years later.

Finally, as my multiple allergic reactions escalated, my local dentist expressed concern for potential sensitivity to the alloy used in this type of crown. I again "dug my teeth in" and researched the use of dental alloys containing titanium. What I found is alarming. According to a study conducted by *Biomedical Engineering News*, "the integrity of restorative dentistry devices containing titanium may be compromised because of the galvanic corrosion problem." The study was designed to measure direct galvanic or coupled corrosion properties of dental restorative and implant materials with titanium. Their testing monitored continuous corrosion potential in conjunction with zero-resistance ammetry. In essence, dental work consisting of titanium could be rusting away!

I relate my personal experience, and the results of the study, to illustrate the potential chemical hazard and biochemical reaction of restorative dental work, particularly in persons with MARS and EI. If you have restorative dentistry and your immune system is compromised, consult with a dentist who is biologically-aware, knowledgeable in dealing with chemical sensitivities, and willing to work with your health-care provider. I'm extremely fortunate to have a dentist that "dug" for the cause of my inflammation. The next challenge was finding a replacement for the crown, and a cementing compound with a lower potential for reaction. I had the crowns replaced and had no reactions to the new restoration or the cement. Isn't it unfortunate that our beautiful restorative dental work has the potential to take a "bite" out of our health?

Don't be Numb to Anesthetics

Be sure your dentist is prepared to administer anesthetics that contain **no** preservatives—an area often over-looked, with serious consequences. If you have problems with the preservative-free anesthetic, ask your dentist about safe options for anesthesia (such as I.V. sedation or acupuncture). **Don't assume** he's prepared; discuss your needs with the dentist, **not** a staff member. Chemical responses can be life-threatening and require serious precautions. Don't risk misinterpretation by a third party. Until your body repairs and your tolerance to foreign chemicals lessen, your trip to the dental office will not be the same. You may be confronted with new sensitivities, not evident until you experience a chemical reaction. It would be impossible to predict the outcome of exposure to the many chemicals used in any medical facility, and dentistry is no exception. Remember to consult with your dentist about the seriousness of your sensitivities **before** you need to make the trip to the dental office.

Even lingering chemicals in the air can trigger a reaction. It's best to schedule an appointment first thing in the morning to reduce exposure to a daily build-up of substances. Be sure your dentist and you are both prepared.

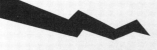

Flash-Back

After developing my allergic responses, my dentist took extraordinary steps to prevent a reaction. Fortunately, he has experience in dealing with these disorders and incorporates a wholistic approach in his practice. Neither one of us knew what to expect.

He protected my face from direct contact to latex, scheduled my appointment first thing in the morning and used minimum local anesthetic with no epinephrine.

During my dental appointment, everything was fine; I had no immediate allergic response. Within an hour of returning home, I developed a pounding headache. At first, I dismissed the symptom. As the day and evening progressed, the headache intensified and became acute. I felt as if my brain was swollen, and my scalp bruised. The next day I had extreme exhaustion. I contacted my dentist, who had already called after office hours to check on me, and I reported the escalating headache. Similar symptoms had been experienced in patients with MARS/EI, so I was quite concerned. He believed the cause was the preservative in the local anesthetic. The headache finally disappeared after two days, while lingering fatigue and light-headedness lasted several more days. For my subsequent dental work, my dentist special-ordered local anesthetic without preservatives or epinephrine to reduce the risk of reacting. I had no reaction to the preservative-free anesthetic. The brand he used is Polocaine™; however, there are several brands available to dentists that meet these protocols.

I was

Poisoned

by my body...

FALSE SENSE OF SECURITY

Two years ago I developed an acute sore throat on the left side when I swallowed. It was relentless. Prior to the sore throat, I enjoyed my usual bountiful energy for traveling, lecturing, teaching, and consulting. I was living what I teach, and felt great. You can image my old "fear" of past memories that emerged—suddenly I was tired all the time, fibromyalgia symptoms returned, dark circles appeared under my eyes, my elimination became sluggish, and the sore throat eventually became a defined swollen gland under the chin. After repeated visits and testing with my conventional physician, all that was echoed was "everything is within normal range"—I then knew it was time again to employ all my expertise as a "health detective," see my dentist and insist we investigate further.

My lower left molars were crowned in gold in 1966. In spite of no dental pain and the x-rays not showing any decay, abscess or inflammation, I knew we had to look beneath the lower left crowns. With hesitation, at my insistence, my dentist removed the crown on the first molar on the lower left

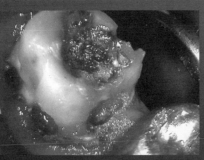

and the following is what he uncovered—I wish I had a picture of the expression on his and his assistant's face!

I was again being poisoned, this time by an exposed root from rampant decay under my crown which did not show on x-rays. The tooth was built-up using a mercury amalgam filling and the poisons were pouring directly into my blood—no wonder I had a one-sided sore throat that felt like a knife was piercing every time I swallowed! If you look closely at the photo, you see the exposed nerve and the shiny mercury at the edge (for color photos see my website at www.gloriagilbere.com).

Flash-Forward (cont.)

The tooth was extracted and replaced by a bridge. Even though I had worked in dentistry, I forgot amalgams were used in that era to build a weakened tooth structure to prepare it for a crown. Don't become a victim of false security just because you've had your amalgam fillings replaced with crowns…the clues to your invisible illness could be lurking under your expensive dental restorations, mine was.

Find a biologically-aware dentist and discuss your medical history and symptoms before any work is performed. The optimum protocol is to have your dentist work with someone like myself to design a protocol for detoxification to reduce your overall toxic load before dental restorations or surgery is performed.

My physician suggested antibiotics—even though no clear evidence of infection was present. Had I agreed, they would compromise intestinal integrity and provide opportunistic entry for *Candida* yeast and, again, the decline of my overall immune system.

Once the infection was identified and the tooth extracted, I took a unique type of silver hydrosol, Argentyn 23™, that is available only from health-care professionals. This patented process, and silver hydrosol in general, has historically been used against viruses, bacteria, fungi, infections, allergies, as nature's immune support and antibiotic alternative, and as a tissue regeneration catalyst. For complete details about the historical use of silver for immune protection, its health benefit, the science behind silver, and answers to the most asked questions about silver in health care, refer to the E-Guide available on my website at www.gloriagilbere.com.

The silver I discuss in the E-Guide is Sovereign Silver™, available over the counter and of the same genre. The silver referred to in this book is a higher potency available only through physicians and practitioners.

(cont. on next page)

I was

Poisoned

by my body…

Flash-Forward (cont.)

Additionally, I supported my immune system with a professional plant sterol product called Sterol 117®. This natural supplement acts as an immune modulator—stimulating a sluggish immune system, calming an over-stimulated one.

I took five capsules once a day during my dental health challenges and continue to take one-two a day for year-around protection (see Resources). It is best taken first thing in the morning after all-night fasting, and then wait 30-45 minutes before consuming anything except water. It especially should *not* be taken with dairy products. I take it upon arising, do my workout, shower, and then have my herbal coffee—an easy way to fit it into my busy schedule.

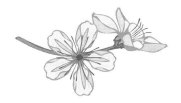

How Did I Get This Way?
Identifying Causes = Power

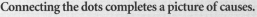

Flash-Back

Connecting the dots completes a picture of causes.
I had a history of chronic constipation and migraine headaches since childhood because of challenging personal situations, the conventional medical diagnosis was always the same: "stress induced." Through natural health care and the emotional support of my paternal grandmother, I successfully overcame these debilitating conditions. Symptoms of constipation did not reappear until decades later when injuries from my life-threatening fall necessitated taking prescription medications. As a result of the accident, I was hospitalized and placed in intensive care. I developed blood clots, pulmonary embolism, and was administered oral and I.V. medications to thin my blood. During my stay in the intensive care unit, I was prescribed medications for pain, inflammation, and muscle relaxation.

When I entered the hospital I had no muscle pain or fatigue and enjoyed a high level of energy and stamina. I had a successful practice, including occupational and natural health care, and enjoyed good quality of life. Shortly after my release from the hospital, I developed what was diagnosed as chronic fatigue. The doctors attributed my symptoms to trauma recuperation. Little did I know this would begin a health-depleting vicious cycle.

(cont. on next page)

I was

Poisoned

by my body...

Flash-Back (cont.)

As my complaints grew in intensity, so did the list of prescribed drugs for symptom-care. I was prescribed antidepressant drugs (benzodiazepines), because I was apparently too impatient to regain my energy and stamina, anti-inflammatory drugs because of muscle pain and decreasing pain tolerance, and muscle relaxing drugs because of my inability to sleep.

The diagnosis of fibromyalgia followed based on my soft and connective tissue pain and accompanying chronic insomnia. I was told that because I was "under excessive stress" I developed fibromyalgia. You bet I was under stress! I had very little quality of life. I could only work four hours a day instead of the usual twelve. I was sleep-deprived and my body was so sore it felt like the nerve endings were on top of my skin. I looked fine on the outside; my maladies were invisible manifestations of internal damage. How could this pain and frustration be explained to the observer when everything external looked normal?

My odyssey continued until I determined no one was getting to the causes; precisely why clients seek my guidance. We were merely causing more and more drug side-effects which became drug-management.

I finally took back charge of my own health and regained a quality of life through alternative therapies with only minor residues of past symptoms from unsuspected exposures. I proceeded completing a Ph.D. in Natural Health and presented my thesis, "Fibromyalgia, known causes, effects and cures, using a Natural Approach." What followed became my encouragement to write this book as described in "My Story."

What Function Does the Gut Perform?

The function of the gastrointestinal tract (GI), or gut, is complex.

Basically, it:

• digests foods

- carries nutrients (vitamins and minerals) attached to carrier proteins across the gut lining into the blood supply
- functions as a major component of the body's detoxification system
- contains immunoglobulins (antibodies)—functioning as the first line of defense against infection

Gut Heath = Overall Health

The gut performs the job of a human chemical factory. It contains billions of intestinal bacteria that have an important effect on human physiology. They produce toxins and anti-toxins that alter the chemical composition of foods and drugs. The number of bacteria in the large intestine (colon) is estimated to be one hundred billion—cells in the entire human body are estimated to be between 50-100 trillion. Intestinal bacteria perform vital functions by keeping the digestion and assimilation of consumed substances in balance. In leaky gut syndrome (LGS), the intestinal lining allows substances and bacteria to leak through into the circulatory system, triggering the body's allergic responses in its attempt to warn of danger.

LGS is caused by inflammation of the intestinal lining, characterized by damage to individual cells. The damaged cells are less able to produce enzymes and other healthy secretions necessary for effective digestion and absorption of nutrients.

The intestines contain some of the most toxic organisms imaginable (bacteria, fungus, yeast overgrowth, toxic residue from chemicals, bile salts, and parasites), known to be responsible for the breakdown of the immune system. Healthy functioning intestines keep these substances normalized, (in control), and prevent them from leaking into circulation.

When leakage of "bad" bacteria occurs, they enter and surround the connective tissue, creating inflammatory responses. As a result of this inflammation and cell damage, the white blood cells (our Pac-man scavengers of abnormal bacteria) must deal with excessive antigen overload. Preoccupied with this task; the cells are prevented from performing effective clean-up.

Destruction of Health *Begins* in the Colon

Allow me to take you on a trip through the gastrointestinal tract, or food canal, of the human body.

Ignoring technical anatomical details, the food canal is a sequence of muscular tubes about ten times the length of the body, measured from the top of the head to the end of the spinal column. The circular muscles of the lips control the upper end of the canal, which is evident when whistling. The mouth and teeth prepare food to undergo the varied processes performed within deeper parts. Circular muscles at various other locations along the canal regulate movements of foodstuffs during the digestion process. The small intestine is coiled up in the lower cavity of the trunk below the diaphragm.

At the lower end of the canal is the colon, wonderfully designed to receive and discharge unused remnants of food and other waste from the body. The colon is sacculated, meaning it is formed from a series of connected pouches, unlike the small intestine with its smooth tube of uniform size.

At the extreme lower end of the canal is the anus, controlled by circular muscles that act voluntarily and involuntarily. Both in health and disease these "food gates" have an important relation to digestion and elimination.

Respected medical authorities understood the importance of colon health since the late 19th century. In this century, the vital role of colon health was generally ignored. Practitioners of natural medicine, and some nutritionally aware physicians, are again validating its vital contribution to the disease processes. Modern studies of the colon show that by neglect, this temporary reservoir of wastes becomes a veritable breeding place of disease and disorders, many described as "incurable." Professor Keith, an eminent English anatomist, attributes diseases of the colon to the adoption of a diet unsuited to human anatomy. Therefore, we are not only what we eat, we are the total sum of how we digest and eliminate what we consume.

The colon forms a receptacle for wastes and excretory substances, together with unusable or undigested residues of food and drugs. The collection of waste is only an incidental function of the colon; its most important function is to conduct these unusable materials out of the body as fecal wastes.

Constipation

There are many causes of constipation; however, for the purposes of this book, I'll discuss those related to LGS and the consequences of prescription drug therapies.

Do you know?...

✓ Americans spend $750,000,000 a year on laxatives.

✓ Physicians write more than 1,200,000 prescriptions annually for constipation medications.

✓ Nearly every man, woman, and child living in a westernized society today is constipated.

✓ A misconception exists that if you eliminate once a day, you are normal and healthy. Consider this: if you eat three meals a day, and eliminate once (or less) daily, where is the rest being stored? Often, the whole length of the five-foot colon is completely packed with old hardened matter, creating a narrow channel for eliminating only small soft feces, or small compressed matter, to pass. This condition is commonly referred to as "tunnel elimination." In other words, fecal matter accumulates on the walls of the colon and eventually attaches, causing the canal of elimination to narrow.

✓ Victims of chronic diarrhea also suffer a form of constipation as a result of narrowing passage ways from colonic plaque, restricting elimination to liquids or matter soft or small enough to pass. This condition is not describing diarrhea as a result of food or water-borne bacteria, but rather from constipation.

To better understand the meaning of the word "constipate," look at its origin. The Latin origin is *constipare*, meaning to press together or compact. Therefore, constipation is a condition in which the feces are packed or pressed together. There are three types of constipation, detailed in the following sections.

Common Constipation

This condition exists when feces passing from the body are overly dry, packed together, and elimination of bowel content is incomplete. Eliminations can be two or more times daily with no additional symptoms. This condition usually results from lack of dietary fiber, processed foods, irregular eating schedules, lack of hydration, and neglecting the urge to eliminate. Typical American diets consist of less than 12 grams of fiber. Recommendations of fiber intake for proper colon health are 20-35 grams daily—without these amounts the colon is unable to brush fecal material from the colon walls. This condition can generally be corrected by increasing dietary fiber, taking the time for regular eliminations, and increasing water consumption. Water is vital in providing sufficient hydration to facilitate elimination; its importance cannot be overstated.

Concealed Constipation

This type of constipation typically occurs in people suffering from chronic disease. Concealed constipation takes years to develop and most people are not aware of its presence because the bowels move daily. Symptoms of this kind of constipation include unexplained fatigue, headaches, bad breath, chronic appendicitis, colitis, PMS, anxiety, and depression. The long-term effects are not recognized until secondary symptoms or disorders emerge. More often than not, this constipation is accelerated by lack of exercise, commonly brought on by pain and discomfort from chronic disease or disorders like fibromyalgia, chronic fatigue, arthritis, long-term use of prescribed medications, and excessive consumption of alcohol and illegal drugs.

Drug-Induced Constipation

Drug-induced constipation is a potentially serious type, as was my case after my accident from consuming pain medications, symptoms generally manifesting within a few days of taking a medication. Drug-induced constipation, in combination with concealed constipation, is a sure prescription for LGS. This constipation occurs particularly with high-potency painkillers, antacids with aluminum, iron supplements, most narcotics, anti-anxiety and anti-depressant medications, especially drugs in the benzodiazepine genre.

The following are examples of commonly prescribed drugs for inflammation, pain, insomnia, depression, and anxiety, with constipating side-effects in most people:

- Hydrocodone/APAP®
- Acetaminophen with codeine
- Naproxen®
- Alprazolam®
- Lorazepam®

- Valium®
- Prednisone®
- Amitriptyline®
- Trazodone®
- Halcion®
- Xanax®

Laxatives: Short Term Solution, Long Range Impact

Laxatives are employed to give immediate bowel relief—they merely stimulate the bowel to move. Chronic use causes the bowel to become lazy and muscles to become dependent on them to constrict. Taking laxatives is *not* a substitute for fiber, water consumption and exercise. Most laxatives irritate the colon, causing damage to colon walls and nerve cells, and forcing the bowels to expel the laxative and anything else loose enough to flow. This action generally makes no specific attempt to expel anything older than the laxative itself—it *does not* dislodge stagnant material within the colon. For this reason, laxatives are a quick fix with no real colon-cleansing benefits. Once the laxative passes through the colon, you're right back where you started (with a plugged-up sewer system) and now you've created irritation from the laxative along with depletion of minerals and health-enhancing bacteria.

If you use laxatives for prolonged periods of time, you'll need to re-train your body to eliminate without the laxative "crutch." Don't ignore your body's urge to defecate, take the time. Regular elimination is imperative to good health. The longer the waste stays in the body, the more toxic material is available to enter the blood supply.

Flash-Forward

After using several herbal supplement stool softeners, I found a product that does not contain herbs known to be habit-forming like Cascara Sagrada or Senna, yet encourages hydration and evacuation. The product is EliminAid™.

Keep in mind fiber loosens colonic plaque; herbs in the stool softener facilitate softening, encourage peristalsis and hydration to flush loosened matter—providing complete evacuation. You should always consume plenty of dietary fiber and supplements that are vegetable fiber colon cleansing blends. However, if you are plagued with constipation of any kind, the use of an herbal stool-softener is a healthy addition to your fiber and colon-cleansing protocol (see Resources).

I now only need to take EliminAid™ along with my fiber supplement when traveling because of reduced water consumption, change in daily routine, and long periods of sitting. I take one capsule at the same time as my fiber caplets anytime in the late afternoon or evening.

Helpful Drugs—Serious Side-Effects

Non-steroidal Anti-inflammatory Drugs (NSAIDs)

NSAIDs are non-steroidal drugs, as distinguished from those that contain corticosteroids. They are a group of drugs frequently used to reduce swelling, inflammation, pain, and fever. The drugs work by inhibiting cyclooxygenase—the enzyme responsible for the production of prostaglandins, hormone-like substances involved in the development of pain and inflammation.

The following statistics regarding use of NSAIDs are alarming, especially considering they only account for annual amounts in the U.S.

✓ 75 million prescriptions for NSAIDs are written annually.

✓ 7,600 people die from gastrointestinal bleeding and perforation—one death for every 9,210 prescriptions.

✓ 76,000 are hospitalized—one hospitalization for every 921 prescriptions.

✓ $100 million are spent annually on gastrointestinal ulcers alone.

✓ *Medical Advertising News* estimates 20,000 deaths each year are attributed to NSAID-induced complications, and the number is rapidly growing.

According to the medical journal *Lancet*, chronic use of NSAIDs, especially in high doses, increases permeability (leaking) of the colon. This leaking actually creates allergies and contributes to arthritic and inflammatory symptoms, the very reason most people take NSAIDs in the first place. This category of drugs comes in many forms—prescription and many over-the-counter formulations.

The most commonly used NSAIDs include, but are not limited to:

Non-Steroidal Anti-Inflammatory Drugs (NSAIDs)

- Ibuprofen®
- ASA
- Indomethacin®
- Aspirin
- Actron®
- Advil®
- Aleve®
- Ketroprofen®
- Motrin®
- Naprosine®
- Naproxen® Sodium
- Teleprin®

RxLists of Indications and Side-Effects reports the following common side-effects associated with NSAID use:

- Abdominal pain
- Diarrhea
- Agranulocytosis
- Dizziness
- Amblyopia
- Drowsiness
- Anemia
- Dyspepsia
- Angioedema
- Dyspnea
- Anorexia
- Edema
- Aplastic anemia
- Elevated hepatic enzymes
- Azotemia
- Bleeding
- Erythema nodosum
- Blurred vision
- Exfoliative dermatitis
- Bronchospasm
- Flatulence
- Bullous rash
- Gastritis
- Cholestasis
- GI bleeding
- Constipation
- GI perforation
- Corneal deposits
- Granulocytopenia

- Headache
- Hearing loss
- Heart failure
- Hematuria
- Hemolysis
- Hepatic failure
- Hepatitis
- Hyperkalemia
- Hypertension
- Hyperuricemia
- Infection
- Insomnia
- Interstitial nephritis
- Intraventricular
  disorder
- Hemorrhage
- Jaundice
- Keratitis
- Lethargy
- Leukopenia
- Maculopapular rash
- Malaise
- Melena
- Musculoskeletal
  inflammation
- Nausea/vomiting
- Nephrotic syndrome
- Occult GI bleeding
- Ocular irritation
- Osteoarthritis
- Palpitations
- Pancreatitis
- Pancytopenia
- Peptic ulcer
- Peripheral edema
- Photosensitivity
- Platelet dysfunction
- Proteinuria
- Pruritus
- Pseudoporphyria
- Purpura
- Renal papillary necrosis
- Retinal hemorrhage
- Reye's syndrome
- Rheumatoid arthritis
- Seizures
- Stevens-Johnson
  syndrome
- Tachycardia
- Tendonitis
- Thrombosytopenia
- Tinnitus
- Toxic epidermal
  necrolysis
- Urticaria
- Vasculitis
- Vertigo
- Visual impairment

Steroidal Drugs

Prescription corticosteroids, including prednisone, are commonly used for inflammatory disorders. Use of steroidal drugs is known to contribute to yeast overgrowth in the digestive system and liver damage.

Acetaminophen (Tylenol®)

Acetaminophen products, like Tylenol, aren't a classic NSAID; however, more than other classes of pain-relief medications, they do induce some of the same effects and appear to be closely related to NSAIDs. Tylenol® does not specifically appear to affect prostaglandins. However, keep in mind that extended use or large doses of acetaminophen can lead to liver damage and, with LGS and most digestive disorders, the liver function is already compromised.

Over-the-Counter (OTC) Pain Relievers

Stronger NSAIDs require a prescription, but lower-dose NSAIDs, such as formulations containing ibuprofen, are available as OTC preparations and are often *thought* to be relatively safe by consumers. How many times have you, or someone you know, taken an ibuprofen to relieve pain, stiffness and/or swelling? You take these medications regularly, perhaps even daily, without much thought of the impending consequences. After all, "They're available without my doctor's prescription, so they can't be too harmful." Anti-inflammatory drugs such as aspirin, ibuprofen, and many over-the-counter drugs are not harmless. They're drugs!

Dozens of OTC medications for pain and inflammation may initially appear to be much less likely to upset the stomach lining than stronger prescription drugs; however, they are just as damaging to the intestinal lining. They are still NSAIDs and cause damage to the lining by blocking the prostaglandin stimulating tissue repair processes. *Keep in mind that while NSAIDs act as anti-inflammatories in the blood-stream and body tissues, they have an irritant or caustic effect in the gastrointestinal tract and damage the lining of the microvillus in the intestinal wall. NSAIDs are a direct cause of LGS and can lead to food and environmental-response syndromes and inflammatory disorders, as in my case.* The consumer may not initially experience the resulting damage or irritation to the colon and digestive system. Consumers are overwhelmed dealing with the symptoms of pain and inflammation and concerned with immediate relief. If NSAID side-effects are suspected, the consumer commonly looks for the most common, quick, old-fashioned solution—aspirin for pain and antacids for GI distress, adding insult to injury.

Aspirin

It is common in today's society to take an aspirin for a headache, to calm down pain of arthritis or fibromyalgia, or to get rid of all those body aches after a day of gardening, shopping or driving. The Aspirin Foundation boasts that this chemical "has probably been taken, at one time or another, by almost every human being on earth." Americans gulp down an estimated 40 million doses of aspirin per day—no wonder digestive disorders and multiple allergic responses are escalating exponentially.

Americans are not alone in their over-indulgence of aspirin. While in Europe, I was amazed to observe the quantities and forms being used *as if* a healthy daily nutritional supplement—in Britain as powdered forms, in France as rectal suppositories, in Germany topical creams, and in Spain effervescents.

Chemical companies produce over 100 million aspirin tablets a year. Consumers are bombarded with commercial and professional advice to consume "an aspirin a day" to prevent heart attacks. *The Physician's Health Study* reported that the preventive aspect of aspirin used for clinical studies was a buffered form containing magnesium as in Bufferin®. Researchers reported that the magnesium component, not the aspirin, is the specific protector of the heart. Magnesium is necessary for every cell in the body—it dilates blood vessels, aids absorption of potassium into the cells (preventing heartbeat irregularities), and assists in keeping blood cells from sticking together (thrombosis). Autopsies of the heart muscle, following death by heart attack, almost always reveal the heart muscle is deficient in magnesium.

A British study using *plain aspirin* revealed aspirin may lower the incidence of heart attack by the anti-coagulant (blood thinning) effect. However, it was not reported that every time you take aspirin you bleed a little into the gut. A microscope will show blood in fecal matter of anyone on daily aspirin. If it's happening in your intestinal tract, how do you know it's not happening in your brain? Doesn't it make you wonder what else might be precipitated by chronic aspirin intake? It makes me question how many fatal hemorrhages of the brain, spleen, liver, intestine, or lung occur after an accident, because the blood has been thinned by excessive aspirin consumption. Many of my clients, as well as me, are being advised by their physicians to take daily doses of aspirin, especially after an accident like mine resulting in thrombosis (blood clots). Additionally, many seniors are advised to take aspirin daily as a preventive measure against diseases associated with aging.

It is alarming to sit on my side of the health-care desk and listen to the long list of symptoms associated with regular aspirin consumption. When clients make the decision to stop the daily aspirin routine, many of their symptoms disappear. For example, during a routine health assessment consultation, a client will describe occasional rectal bleeding. When symptoms of rectal bleeding are reported to their physician during routine check-ups, the medical rectal exams show no evident cause (polyps, hemorrhoids, etc.). However, when I inquire about aspirin consumption, most answer, "Yes, daily, I've been told it's good for me." When clients decide to stop the aspirin for a trial period, they report no rectal bleeding occurred during the test period. When they resume daily intake of aspirin, rectal bleeding is again evident. This tells me a lot, and it should send up red flags for you, too!

What is even more alarming are findings published in the *British Medical Journal*. The journal reported the conclusions of California researchers: older men and women who take aspirin every day double their risk of developing ischemic heart disease, the very disease they were attempting to prevent. Ischemic heart disease accounts for a wide range of symptoms caused by blockage of cardiac arteries. The study also found that aspirin users were more likely to develop kidney and colon cancer. These studies, as well as personal and professional experience, make me question how many other disorders might have started from the use of aspirin. Maybe for many of us, aspirin began the "gut reaction" of intestinal disorders—a thought worth digesting.

Prescription Pain Medications

MEDICATIONS FOR PAIN AND INFLAMMATION = DAMAGE TO INTESTINAL LINING = PAIN AND INFLAMMATION

The pain may be reduced temporarily with the use of pain medications, however, their toxic effects of tissue and/or organ damage are yet to manifest as a disease or disorder—generally constipation, heartburn, LGS and overgrowth of *Candida* yeast.

As earlier described, constipation is a serious side-effect of many pain medications, especially codeine-containing drugs such as hydrocodone/APAP.

Flash-Forward

I now take several natural complexes when I develop pain or inflammation, usually from consuming unsuspected nightshade foods or from too many hours at my computer without my usual stretch breaks on my rebounder. Elsewhere in this book I describe the supplements I use and recommend that are extremely effective without the dangerous side-effects previously discussed.

Stress and Your Digestive System

Stresses do not directly cause LGS or associated digestive disorders; however, they contribute to development of disorders because excessive or prolonged stress lowers the body's overall resistance.

Dr. Hans Selye, known for his research related to stress, refers to inflammatory diseases as one of the "stress diseases." Adrenal exhaustion from prolonged stress is one of the major causes leading to the development of inflammatory and digestive disorders.

The pituitary and/or adrenal glands, after prolonged stress and consequent impaired metabolism, are no longer able to function normally to produce cortisone, desoxycortisone, aldosterone, and other naturally occurring hormones. This impaired metabolism results in severe hormonal imbalances, further metabolic derangement, and lowered resistance to stress from infections, drugs, and toxic substances in food and the environment. According to famed nutritionist, the late Adele Davis, "Meeting the demands of stress should be your first consideration." The best way to accomplish this is to adopt a self-care life-style of eating a nutrient rich diet of organic un-processed fresh vegetables, fruits, grains, and seeds, and insuring your environment is as free of toxic chemicals as possible.

Stress plays a major role in digestive disorders—sustained stress in our mind, body, and spirit affects its ability to heal. One of the body's reactions to stress is the slowing of digestion and reduction of blood flow to digestive organs—straining the gastrointestinal tract's ability to function at full capacity.

Candida (Systemic Yeast Overgrowth) = Dysbiosis

Your Internal Ecosystem

Just as the forest must have enough vegetation to filter toxins in the environment, our body needs to contain an abundance of "friendly" health-enhancing bacteria to balance the "unfriendly" health-depleting ones. Nowadays, our intestinal ecosystems are subjected to sugars, refined foods, antibiotics, corticosteroids and barrages of drugs that disturb or destroy our intestinal balance.

Dysbiosis Defined

Dysbiosis was a term coined by Dr. Eli Metchnikoff in the early 1900s. He won the Nobel Prize in 1908 for his work on lactobacilli (health-enhancing bacteria) and their role in immunity. He was a colleague of Louis Pasteur and succeeded him as director of the Pasteur Institute in Paris. The origin of the term "dysbiosis" came from the word "symbiosis," which means to live together in mutual harmony. Dysbiosis was derived from the original term by the prefix "dys," meaning not—dysbiosis is an unbalanced intestinal tract. In a healthy, balanced intestinal terrain, health-enhancing microorganisms combat overgrowth of yeast, fungi, parasites, and health-depleting bacteria.

Candidiasis (Candida)

The most common form of dysbiosis is *Candida*, a fungal infection. *Candida* is a normally occurring fungus living in the mucous membranes, especially in the digestive tract and vagina. It is also found in the sinuses, ear canals,

Photo used with permission by Victoria Glassburn, author of *Who Killed Candida?*

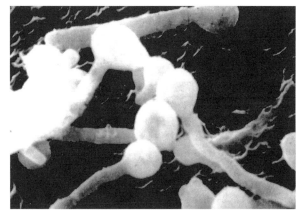

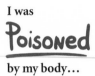
and genitourinary tract. The healthy body can handle normal amounts of this fungus—in large amounts, it contributes to the decline of digestive health. In healthy conditions, *Candida* yeast organisms live in harmony with other organisms within the intestines. When the immune system is weakened, it encourages *Candida* growth. When yeast outnumbers other bacteria (*Candida albicans* overgrowth), the condition is called "Candidiasis."

Causes of Candida

There are multiple causes facilitating this yeast to grow out of control. Our western civilization is accustomed to a diet of fast and convenient foods, rich in sugar, yeast, additives and preservatives. The extensive use of antibiotics also results in yeast overgrowth. Antibiotics destroy both health-enhancing and health-depleting bacteria. Yeast is *not* killed by antibiotics, but rather flourishes in the resulting *imbalance* of intestinal bacteria. After antibiotic therapy is complete, the reduced population of health-enhancing bacteria encourages yeast to multiply at alarming rates. *Candida* overgrowth, in turn, releases toxic by-products that add to the already weakened immune system. In the case of LGS, the already weakened immune system now has the added toxins leaking through intestinal walls.

- Extreme fatigue
- Lethargy
- Foggy thinking
- Depression
- Yeast infections
- Poor memory
- Mood swings
- Muscle weakness
- Multiple allergies
- Athlete's foot
- Nail fungus
- Bloating and gas
- Nasal congestion
- Post-nasal drip
- Vinegar cravings
- Skin fungus infections
- Jock itch
- Carbohydrate cravings
- Sugar cravings
- Unexplained anxiety
- Blood sugar imbalances
- Chronic fatigue
- Heightened symptoms in damp, muggy, moldy places
- Sensitivities to cigarette, perfume, fabric odors
- Generalized environmental sensitivities
- Recurring sinus and ear infections

Few health-care providers are aware that many of today's disorders are yesterday's yeast. It's my experience that you don't see a person with LGS without systemic yeast overgrowth, and most people with excessive yeast overgrowth have LGS to some degree.

Parasitic Involvement—
"What's Bugging You?"

Yes, I know this will open a "can of worms," however, parasites and abnormal bacteria irritate the intestinal lining—contributing to intestinal disorders. Parasites are opportunistic invaders; when the intestinal and immune system is in healthy balance, there is less opportunity for parasitic infestation. Antibiotics for parasitic infestations are not a viable option; they kill bacteria indiscriminately, health-enhancing and disease-causing bacteria, disrupting the intestinal ecosystem. Patients with compromised immunity and/or low fiber intake are at greater risk for opportunistic infections.

Parasites and worms are scavenger organisms living within, upon, or at the expense of a host organism, without contributing to the survival of the host (you). They reside in the gastrointestinal tract and feed on toxins and waste in the body. The most common are roundworms (hookworms, pinworms, and threadworms) and tapeworms. The danger of these uninvited visitors is the waste materials expelled into the host body—extremely toxic, even deadly, and are associated with many diseases.

Unfortunately, most medical professionals never suspect parasitic infections, and when conventional testing is performed, seldom confirm their presence if they're not specifically within that specimen. Parasites are generally associated with AIDS, colon disorders, some types of cancer, chronic fatigue syndrome, irritable bowel syndrome, psoriasis, and *Candida*. Frequent use of antibiotics, a diet low in fiber and high in sugar, and many prescription medications, reduce beneficial intestinal flora, providing a nourishing environment for parasites and worms to flourish. If you have a chronic digestive condition that resists treatment and the onset of symptoms occurred after a trip to specifically, but not limited to, Central or South America, Asian-Pacific countries, Africa, Oceania, under-developed countries, or the Middle-East, you most likely have parasitic involvement. These examples are not to imply that only these regions of the world carry parasitic risks, rather presented as the relationship between travel and chronic disorders that manifest after a trip out of the U.S. Many experts believe there are as many parasitic infestations within the U.S. in recent years as in other parts of the world. I agree.

One common type of infection, giardiasis, is so common in some areas that the entire population hosts this microorganism. Also known as "Travelers Diarrhea," "Montezuma's Revenge," "Delhi Belly," "Turistas" and "GI Trots," this condition causes violent cramping and diarrhea that continues despite the use of over-the-counter medications. *Giardia* organisms are regularly found in mountain streams. More alarming is the fact they infect many of our city water systems, since *Giardia is not killed by chlorina-*

tion. Water is the main avenue for spread of giardiasis in the U.S. and abroad. For the past several years, the Center for Disease Control (CDC) has reported that *Giardia* organism is the most prevalent cause of waterborne disease in America. According to the Environmental Protection Agency (EPA), outbreaks in treated municipal water are doubling approximately every three years.

Symptoms of giardiasis may last for weeks, months, or longer—masquerading for years as other disorders. Recent references in scientific literature suggest this parasitic infestation may be the primary cause of allergies and immune-system disorders, even cancer. Additional research continues to determine just how large a role parasites play. What we do know is they're capable of causing damage to the lining of the digestive tract, allowing large molecules to enter circulation-causing LGS.

Many physicians request generalized parasitology testing on random stool samples; however, this type of testing is not very accurate. It's my experience that the most accurate testing is done by labs specializing in parasitology or tropical medicine, requiring two or more samples and interpreted by specialists.

Flash-Forward

My individualized non-drug protocols have been successful for the elimination of parasites—each designed with attention to the tolerance and overall health of the client. I urge you to seek the counsel of a natural health professional; do not assume one product or protocol is effective and safe for everyone. I use and recommend a combination of a homeopathic parasite remedy and Zymex II®—a professional enzyme blend available only through health professionals.

Colon therapists and clients report amazing results that cannot be denied when they see the organisms being expelled with their own eyes—I'll spare you photos clients send me! That said, for best results, a parasite cleanse should be used along with a broad spectrum colon fiber cleanse product, assisting removal of dead parasites by "brushing" them for rapid elimination.

It is very rare that my clients with MARS or EI do not also have parasite involvement. Many times at my insistence, after regaining some quality of life but not completely symptom-free, they agree to a parasite detoxification protocol—the men are the most challenging to convince. When they finally make the commitment to the protocol, I always get a phone call or email sharing the results with me and wanting to know what they can do to avoid being reinfected. Generally, their allergic responses, allergies, and skin disorders are either dramatically improved or eliminated altogether.

As a course of maintenance, I follow and recommend parasite cleanses for two weeks every six months, after the initial personalized protocol. It's easy, doesn't cause any change to your daily schedule and prevents "uninvited guests." After you experience the results, as my clients and I have, you won't hesitate; you'll wish you'd done it sooner.

How Did I Get
This Way?
Identifying
Causes = Power

Identifying the Problem– Uncovering What Conventional Diagnosis Does *Not*

Innovative Alternative Testing

THE TESTS LISTED BELOW are not ordinary tests performed at your local medical laboratory or hospital. However, more and more laboratories are offering these optional tests as demand increases. Your health-care practitioner or nutritionally-aware physician will be familiar with these innovative testing methods. These laboratories offer complete information packages and test kits, and offer your physician assistance in interpreting the results.

Live Cell Variable Projection Microscopy

This test pioneered the concept of Oxidology, the study of reactive oxygen toxic species (ROTS), in health and disease, as a precise medical sub-specialty. Bradford Research Institute has the most advanced variable projection multi-phase optical microscopy system available. This instrument has made possible the correlation of pathology with the dynamics of peripheral blood morphology, yielding unique insights into clinical and sub-clinical mechanisms.

Live cell analysis is a unique and innovative way to obtain a screening perspective of the amount and general location of the oxidative processes at work within the body, as well as hormones, enzymes and other by-products of biological stresses. Diseases demonstrated are often chronic. However, progressive, acute, sub-acute and degenerative conditions are visible as well. This unique analysis has the ability, among other things, to reveal the condition of the immune system. Some of the constituents clearly observed is the activity of white blood cells; extent of foreign antigens and microbes within the serum; and the strength, condition and movement of red blood cells. These three major components judge the strength of the immune system and might possibly indicate progressive disease processes at work.

A second series of drops is placed on a second slide taken from the same finger prick at the same time, and allowed to dry. This gives further insight into the general location within the body of pathological activity, particular processes, toxin build up, and length of time it has been present.

This type of analysis acts as an educational "feedback mechanism." Changes in the makeup of the blood cells, improvement in toxin amounts, etc. may be viewed periodically as an indicator of progress.

The analysis serves as a barometer for the client and health-care provider, enabling each to monitor health and the changes taking place.

The tests are performed by clinicians and practitioners worldwide and certified by Bradford Research Institute (see how the test is performed in "My Story" and refer to Resources).

Intestinal Permeability Testing

Most of the non-invasive permeability-testing techniques are simple, reliable, and can be used to assess many clinical conditions. This test determines underlying problems linked to GI function. It directly measures how well two non-metabolized sugar molecules, mannitol and lactulose, permeate the intestinal mucosa. Low levels of mannitol and lactulose indicate mal-absorption. Elevated levels of lactulose and mannitol are indicative of general increased permeability and leaky gut syndrome (LGS) phenomena. This test must be ordered by a health-care professional, requires an overnight fast, and can be performed in the privacy of your home (see Resources).

Comprehensive Digestive Stool Analysis (CDSA)

This test evaluates digestion, absorption, intestinal function, and the microbial flora such as *Candida* (yeast overgrowth). The CDSA uncovers the fundamental causes of many acute and chronic symptoms

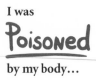
and is used in the evaluation of various gastrointestinal symptoms or systemic illnesses that may have started in the intestines. Because illnesses are often not discernable from symptoms, the CDSA is a valuable means for identifying critical imbalances previously unsuspected (see Resources).

Comprehensive Parasitology Testing

This test can uncover parasitic infections associated with systemic complaints. The diagnosis of most parasitic infections depends on the laboratory. For intestinal parasites, morphological demonstration of diagnostic stages is the principal means of diagnosis. Computer-enhanced video microscopy aids in identification and provides the physician and patient with an actual picture of organisms found (see Resources).

Liver Detoxification Profile

This test assesses the body's capacity to carry out detoxification through functional challenges (caffeine, acetaminophen, and salicylate) which evaluate specific aspects of the detoxification process and free radical damage. These functional assessments provide a comprehensive profile of the body's detoxification capacity and potential susceptibility to oxidative damage. It is a good way to assess the effects of pharmaceutical drugs and herbal substances (see Resources).

Notes:

- *All referenced tests must be ordered by a physician or health-care practitioner. Many of my clients perform parasite elimination protocols without testing, simply because they manifest the symptoms of parasitic infestation and have never performed an in-depth cleanse. If you want scientific photographic proof, spend the money on testing.*

- *Victims of MARS, MCS, and EI cannot always tolerate the substances they are required to consume for testing until initial intestinal toxic load is reduced and liver function improves.*

Identifying the Problem– Uncovering What Conventional Diagnosis Does *Not*

Healing Leaky Gut Naturally–
Not Medicine as Usual

THIS CHAPTER DISCUSSES effective therapies for healing the digestive system. It is advisable to take supplements under the strict guidance of a qualified health-care professional who can suggest the most appropriate course of action for your particular situation. Many people attempting self-treatment, or with the advice of well-meaning sales people without qualified training or experience, do not take the correct products or dosages. Under the guidance of a qualified health professional, you should expect to see some improvement within ninety days. However, it's been my experience, and that of the thousands of clients I've consulted with, that four to six months is necessary for significant reversal of symptoms and improvement in total quality of life. Healing digestive disorders requires a true commitment and life-style change. Considering the options, the majority of my clients and I have chosen the road to recovery via the natural highway.

Strategic Healing

Much has been written about specific protocols for healing leaky gut syndrome (LGS) and the associated disorders. The following recommendations represent the approach that facilitated recovery for my clients and me, repaired LGS, and ultimately reversed MARS and EI—regaining our quality of life. It is **imperative** that you seek counsel from a health-care practitioner who is knowledgeable, successful in working specifically with these disorders, and flexible in mapping the road to recovery to suit your needs.

Systemic Cleaning (Detoxifying)

Therapeutic Functional Foods

Below are three functional foods I most commonly use and recommend for the reasons cited.

1. One of the most effective systemic detoxification products, in my personal and professional experience, is a dietary supplement known as functional food. For supporting the liver and facilitating overall detoxification I use Bio-Cleanse™. It assists the liver in converting an insoluble toxin (hard to remove) to a soluble toxin (easily removed), doing so by assisting the liver's Phase 1 and Phase 2 detoxification pathways. A complex formula, it is designed to support gastrointestinal healing while facilitating the removal of toxic substances from your nervous system, connective and fatty tissues. These toxic substances may be metabolic waste or they may be environmental, such as heavy metals, pesticides, herbicides, solvents, and drug residues, to name a few.

The specialty complex of Bio-Cleanse nutrients is a balanced ratio of protein, carbohydrates, and fats to facilitate the maintenance of healthy blood sugar and energy levels, while also providing a complex of multi-minerals and vitamins. Its base is a hypo-allergenic rice protein concentrate, *free* of most allergens such as wheat, rye, oats, barley, corn, dairy, egg, peanut, artificial colors, fillers, or flavors (available only through health-care professionals, see Resources).

2. Reducing the toxic load is one step on the road to recovery. The second step is providing support nutrients to repair and revitalize gastrointestinal integrity while still supporting liver function. In order to accomplish this, it's important to include nutrients such as glutamine, vegetable derived digestive enzymes, milk thistle, grape seed extract, quercertin, and green tea extract in a micro-nutrient rich, non-GMO rice protein base.

Intestinal RejuvenX™ contains 28 grams of a patented rice protein extract per serving that is easily tolerated by the most sensitive individuals. It provides a "safe" food source for those whose diets are restricted because of multiple allergic responses or chronic illness. It is formulated to specifically promote healthy cholesterol and triglyceride metabolism, healthy regeneration of gastrointestinal cells, and provide multi-minerals and vitamins while selectively promoting growth and replication of health-enhancing microorganisms (available only through health-care professionals, see Resources).

3. Another necessary part of the rejuvenation process is to assist soft and connective tissue repair while reducing inflammation and the resulting pain. BioInflammatory *Plus*™ provides nutrients in therapeutic amounts—not placebo ratios. It is designed to quench inflammation naturally and safely. Inflammatory compounds can be part of the body's own metabolic waste (as in a congested lymphatic system) or they may be the result of environmental toxins, heavy metals, or dental restorations that our body reacts against—a small example of substances capable of causing an allergic response.

BioInflammatory *Plus* provides ingredients to act against free radicals that damage tissues while liberating inflammatory cytokines and prostaglandins in the process. It is designed to reduce inflammatory responses with specialty nutrients and antioxidant-free radical quenchers.

It contains a complex of vitamins, minerals, and specialty nutrients including L-Glutamine and Lysine, Glucosamine Sulfate 2KC1, White Willow bark powder (natural aspirin), Methyl Sulfonyl Methane (MSM), Quercetin, Bromelain, Lemon Bioflavonoids, Papain, N-Acetylcysteine, Trypsin, Chymotrypsin, Serrapeptase, L-Theanine, and provides 15g of protein derived from rice protein concentrate (available only through health-care professionals, see Resources).

Flash-Forward

Dietary changes MUST also be made to avoid foods in the nightshade genre known to accelerate inflammation. For a complete list of foods that create an inflammatory response, you can print a list from my website at no charge.

Clients and readers kept asking for recipe substitutes for nightshades. They also wanted to know the scientific reasons for avoidance and optional nutritional support to medications. I finally completed the book "Pain / Inflammation Matters"—a full-color guide detailing nutritional and supplemental remedies for generalized inflammation, including thirty gourmet recipes to provide you substitutes for inflammation-inducing foods—available for purchase on my website and through major booksellers.

The book details conditions known to have an underlying inflammatory component including heart disease, fibromyalgia, arthritis, lupus, gout, periodontal disorders (gum diseases), and premature aging, to name a few.

Author's Note—The above functional foods are powders that are easily mixed in water, juice, or milk substitute as a base for a protein shake. I always mix mine with water to avoid extra sugars or carbohydrates that feed intestinal yeast. You can use this as a meal substitute or as a nutritious drink anytime. I suggest using functional foods daily as a base during your individual protocol for detoxification and repair. Thereafter, I use and recommend functional foods periodically for maintenance or as needed along with the following nutrients to make a "meal in a glass." You must add, reduce, or subtract ingredients according to your tolerance. If highly sensitive, start with very small amounts, sip slowly and gradually increase.

Gloria's Rejuvenation Protein Shake

2 Scoops (scoop comes in product) Functional
    Food* or 2 TB. Caprotein® goat-milk protein
2 TB. Oil blend of Omega 3, 6 and 9's (Udo's
    Choice®—Oil Blend contains all three)
1 tsp. Organic, Kosher wheatgrass juice concentrates
    (Sheldon Farm®)
1 pkt. Sweet Life™ natural sweetener (or to taste)
2 TB. Goat-milk mineral/electrolyte whey powder
    (Capra Mineral Whey®)

Flash-Forward

* I've used several functional food products—
the above three described are those I currently use and recommend for wellness protocols and periodic maintenance because of their effectiveness and tolerance by those most reactive. That said, if you do not intend to follow an overall detoxification protocol (environmental and intestinal) to reduce your toxic load, and commit for a minimum of ninety days, you will be throwing away money and setting yourself up for failure. These products are effective; they are not a substitute for an in-depth detoxification program that includes reduction of the toxic

Cleansing and Supporting the Lymphatic System

Without our lymphatic system, we could not live. Most people rarely hear about it or understand its complex work except as connected to the disease of cancer as lymphoma.

The lymph system is closely related to the cardio-vascular system, although it's major function in the body is as a defense mechanism. It filters out disease-causing organisms, manufacturers white blood cells, and generates antibodies. It is an important system for the distribution of fluid and nutrients all over the body because it drains off excess fluids and proteins left behind by capillary circulation, preventing tissues from swelling.

The fluid that circulates within the system is called lymph. Derived from blood plasma, although clearer and more watery, lymph seeps through capillary walls to fill tissue spaces. Besides lymph, the system

Flash-Forward (cont.)

load in the colon. They facilitate removal of toxins from various tissues and organs and then provide nutrients for repair—the toxins released still need to be "brushed" and eliminated through the colon before repair can occur.

I now use a similar protein shake daily, and when I travel, I substitute goat-milk protein powder rather than functional food (referenced later in this book)—periodically adding functional food as needed.

includes lymphatic capillaries, larger vessel lymph nodes, glands, spleen, tonsils, and thymus.

Lymph vessels are located throughout the body and are actually more numerous than blood vessels. Lymph is the inner excretory mechanism of the body—four times larger than the blood system and provides the means for each individual cell in the body to get rid of waste. Lymphatic capillaries are vessels scattered throughout the body. Their job is to collect surplus fluid and transport it to two terminal vessel stations. The first, the thoracic duct, is the lymphatic system's main duct, which lies along the spine and enters a large vein on the left, close to the heart. The second, the right lymphatic duct, enters a subclavian vein on the right side.

Substances resulting from cellular metabolism are extruded from the cell and must be removed through the lymph—keeping in mind that lymph is only designed to handle cell wastes. When the blood is also dumping waste toxins from the intestinal tract into the lymph system via the liver, the lymph becomes overworked and its filtering/neutralizing function is decreased.

Lymph and lymphatic vessels come into much more intimate relationships with metabolic tissues than blood. However, unlike the blood system utilizing the heart as a pump, the lymph system, like veins, relies on skeletal muscle contractions to pump its components along.

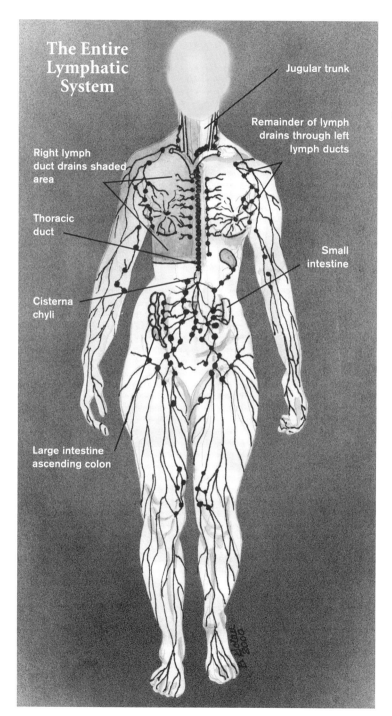

The Entire Lymphatic System

Jugular trunk

Remainder of lymph drains through left lymph ducts

Right lymph duct drains shaded area

Thoracic duct

Small intestine

Cisterna chyli

Large intestine ascending colon

Healing Leaky Gut Naturally— *Not* Medicine as Usual

I was

Poisoned

by my body...

A toxic bowel leaks poisons through smaller veins that gradually join together until they form one large vein, the portal vein, which goes directly to the liver. Lymphatic fluid bathes the tissues in a pale, coagulable fluid. This fluid, riddled with toxins, is then distributed within the blood by way of the thoracic duct. Lymphatic massage, or stimulation as in rebounding, allows excess fluids to flow into the

Hepatic Portal System

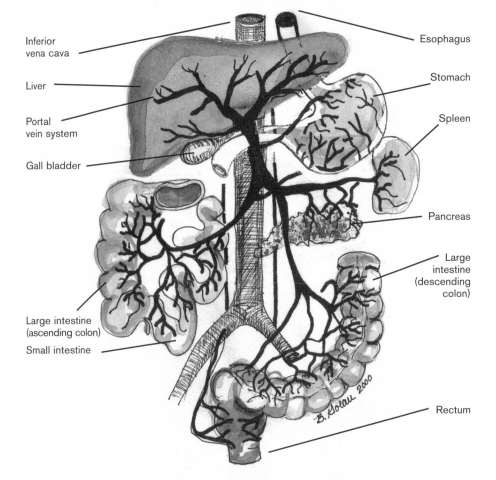

Inferior vena cava

Liver

Portal vein system

Gall bladder

Large intestine (ascending colon)

Small intestine

Esophagus

Stomach

Spleen

Pancreas

Large intestine (descending colon)

Rectum

B. Glotau 2000

lymph filtering stations to flush waste matter—preventing or minimizing escape into the blood supply.

According to nutritionist Robert Gray, stimulating the lymph system with massage allows sticky mucoid toxic substances to be dumped into the colon for elimination, since the colon is the principal organ through which mucoid matter from the lymph is eliminated.

Dr. Loren Berry, one of the greatest of all manipulative healers, taught a technique of lymph drainage using massage therapy, although it was not widely accepted by conventional medical practices at the time.

Dr. Olszewski of Poland conducted studies using scientific instruments capable of stimulating body surfaces by lymphatic massage and skin brushing. His studies concluded that the lymph undergoes *retrograde flow*—flow in the direction *opposite* to that which is considered normal. He also discovered chylous reflux—a specific type of retrograde flow. Chylous reflux occurs when lymph flows from the *cisterna chili* (the central lymphatic pool, in the abdomen) back into the colon or other body tissues. If the colon cannot perform the necessary purification of the lymph, the liver does the work—adding to the toxic load for an already overworked liver.

When toxins are produced in the body at a faster rate than the body can process, the body protects us by suspending those toxins in fat and interstitial spaces in the attempt to protect organs. This excessive amount of toxins results in inflammation and excessive buildup of lymphatic fluids, as in fibromyalgia.

Flash-Back

When my thoracic area was so swollen, it not only caused acute localized pain, it also caused inflammation of the surrounding tissues. The medical diagnosis was "thoracic outlet syndrome." There was no medical explanation for the cause of the swelling or fluid buildup. Anti-inflammatory drug therapy and standard physical therapy was suggested and prescribed. Standard physical therapy brought *no* relief; it included traditional massage and body mechanics, and no specific attention to the lymphatics. After my *first* lymphatic massage, the swelling was gone. It would gradually reoccur and after a lymphatic massage would again disappear. Finally, the body rid itself of enough toxins to facilitate the eventual elimination of swelling and pain.

There are several lymphatic drainage and stimulation techniques. During this stage of my illness, the therapist employed the Loren Berry method. The principles of his technique were developed from ancient Chinese medicine. The lymphatic massage therapist works from the colon to the periphery of the body—from the center out. Space is thus created for the lymph fluid to drain. Undulating hand moves and specific compression is applied to move the fluid while allowing it to be carried through the lymph system and eliminated by the colon—immediately reducing swelling.

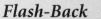

Flash-Back
There came a time when my body let my therapist and me know it no longer could handle a full session (1-1^1/2 hours) of lymph drainage massage. When my body detoxified too quickly, I experienced accelerated fatigue and malaise. Subsequently, my therapist worked only on specific areas, for short periods of time, and with minimum pressure.

You *must* listen to your body, know your limits, and communicate with your therapist. If the massage is too intense, the resulting healing crisis causes you alarm, creates lack of trust in the therapist, and negates benefits of the technique. Our bodies change daily as we detoxify. Have the therapist start slowly with minimum stimulating pressure. Do not allow a therapist to talk you into a deeper massage than you can comfortably tolerate. You'll not only be in pain, but it can trigger an allergic response. For maximum benefit, the therapist must work at your speed to inspire trust, relaxation, and reduction of symptoms. My experiences have proven that deep tissue massage is detrimental for the LGS, MARS, and EI patients because it forces toxins stored in tissue to be quickly released, overworking the organs of detoxification.

Rebounding—Lymph Stimulation and Body "Lift"

Functional foods, supplemental nutrients, and various detoxification and rejuvenation techniques cannot totally repair and maintain health when overall circulation and the lymphatic system are not stimulated to remove toxic residue.

One of the most beneficial exercises I experienced for overall benefits and reduction of fibromyalgia/arthritis symptoms and stagnant lymph flow was, and still is, rebounding. Most victims of disorders that include multiple allergic responses, soft and connective tissue pain, and fatigue, do not have tolerance for exercise. Rebounding works with gravity, rather than against it, protecting against strains and injuries to bones and joints while stimulating lymphatic flow like no other stimulation method can accomplish.

According to Dr. Morton Walker, "rebounding aerobics operates on simple principles. With each gentle bounce, approximately sixty trillion body cells are pitted against the earth's gravitational pull. This interaction strengthens every cell in the body while saving strain on its muscles and joints." Rebounding is an exercise that supports reduction of body fat; firms your legs, thighs, abdomen, arms, and hips; increases agility; improves sense of balance; strengthens muscles; provides an aerobic effect for the heart; rejuvenates your body when it's tired, and generally puts you in a state of health and fitness. A rebounder has extra heavy shock absorbers, unlike a conventional minitrampoline—avoiding injury and stress to joints, especially knees and hips. The following benefits of rebounding are a summary of the health benefits as stated by Dr. Walker in his book *Jumping for Health*:

- ✓ increases capacity for respiration
- ✓ circulates more oxygen to the tissues
- ✓ establishes better equilibrium between oxygen required by tissues and oxygen made available
- ✓ causes muscles to perform work in moving fluids through the body to lighten load on the heart
- ✓ tends to reduce the height to which arterial pressures rise during exertion
- ✓ lessens the time blood pressure remains abnormal after sustained activity
- ✓ delays incidences of cardiovascular disease
- ✓ increases functional activity of red bone marrow in production of red blood cells
- ✓ aids lymphatic circulation, as well as vein flow within the circulatory system
- ✓ encourages collateral circulation
- ✓ strengthens the heart and other muscles so they work more efficiently
- ✓ allows the resting heart to beat less often
- ✓ lowers elevated cholesterol and triglyceride levels
- ✓ stimulates metabolism
- ✓ promotes body growth and repair
- ✓ tones the glandular system—especially encourages thyroid output
- ✓ chemically attains absolute cell potential
- ✓ reserves bodily strength and physical efficiency
- ✓ expands the body's capacity for fuel storage and endurance

✓ improves coordination through the transmission of nerve impulses and responsiveness of muscle fibers

✓ affords muscular vigor from increased muscle fiber tone

✓ offers relief from neck and back pains, headaches, and other pain and stiffness caused by lack of exercise

✓ enhances digestion and elimination processes

✓ allows for better and easier relaxation for enhanced sleep

✓ results in improved mental performance, with keener learning processing

✓ curtails fatigue and menstrual discomfort in women

✓ minimizes the number of colds, allergies, digestive disorders, and abdominal problems

✓ tends to slow aging processes

✓ reduces likelihood of obesity

You can easily perform this exercise in your living room, office, or yard. At first, I only bounced very gently for approximately one minute with my feet never leaving the mat—slowly working up over several weeks to 10 minutes. The swelling in my thoracic and lymph system disappeared within a few days and I slowly regained my stamina and energy.

I've ballroom danced as long as I can remember. Developing these disorders took away the one sport I truly loved that provided exercise for my mind, body, and soul. My whole body was so sore I didn't have

Flash-Forward

Within a year of my illness, I resumed ballroom dancing and was ultimately elected as President of the local chapter of the U.S. Amateur Ballroom Dance Association—a position I was re-elected to for a total of three years.

I now use a rebounder with a stabilizer bar and perform a daily thirty-minute routine to an orchestrated workout or to saucy Latin music—when I don't, my body lets me know it!

After long hours daily at the computer, my rebounder has not only kept my lymph system in good health, it has eliminated muscle fatigue and soreness while toning my body. The benefits of rebounding have been so significant that I incorporated it into my "Wholistic Skin and Body Rejuvenation (WSBR®)" program that I created, guide, and teach around the world. For details about the rebounder I use, and information about my guided rejuvenation programs, visit my website at www.gloriagilbere.com.

the strength to get through even one dance. Rebounding afforded me a "safe" way to regain my strength and stamina in my home and office—free of potential environmental assaults.

Castor Oil Pack—Lymphatic Value

Topical applications of castor oil are recommended by respected physician and researcher, Dr. William McGarey, for disturbances of the digestive system, including stomach, intestines, and colon. He also recommends applications of castor oil for problems of the kidney, liver, and gall bladder. His work, in cooperation with the *Association for Research and Enlightenment*, confirms the use of castor oil for

Flash-Forward

Brain-storming with clients, we finally achieved a method of accomplishing maximum results from castor oil packs. The following describes the technique I use and recommend.

1) Cut a piece of soft cotton cloth from an old sheet, cotton nightwear, or baby diaper (if you can find a cotton one). If you're not extremely sensitive to new fabrics, you can purchase a yard of cotton flannel and wash it several times before using to remove sizing. The size for therapy should be just large enough to cover your abdomen from waist to bottom of torso and side to side.

2) Warm a small amount of castor oil in a glass or stainless steel pan on the cook-top, not microwave.

3) Submerge the cloth in the warm oil, making sure it's saturated but not dripping. Caution: Be sure temperature is bath-water warm, not boiling.

4) Apply the moistened cloth to your abdomen and cover with plastic wrap to maintain heat.

5) After step four, cover the plastic with a warmed dry towel. You may use a heating pad on top of the towel and warm to a comfortable temperature.

6) After the pack cools, you can reheat in pan with additional oil for reuse, or wrap it in plastic wrap then foil, and place in refrigerator to avoid rancidity.

7) The pack can be reused several times and then discarded.

Note: Castor oil stains permanently. Be sure you wear old clothing and protect your furniture and bedding. I used an old pair of sweat pants and shirt and covered my bedding with an old beach blanket.

This procedure is extremely beneficial for reducing cramping, constipation, bloating and pain. It can be safely used anytime, especially right before or after colon hydrotherapy.

disturbances in the lymphatic, circulatory, urinary, and excretory systems. Castor oil has numerous external applications and can be applied by massaging the oil into the skin or by applying castor oil packs. I find castor oil extremely valuable for reducing the inflammation of both the abdominal and liver areas—it encourages activity and movement of lymph fluid through the vessels. By increasing mobility, lymph fluids, fats, and other waste deposits are quickly eliminated. Rebounding, massage stimulation, and application of castor oil encourage circulation of lymph.

According to Dr. McGarey, castor oil absorbed into the tissues stimulates the parasympathetic nerve system in the area being treated. This in turn stimulates the lymphatics to more adequately drain the tissues under stress. Such activity would be beneficial to any organ or portion of the body clogged with waste products.

Skin Brushing—Its Benefits

Skin brushing is a highly effective technique for gently stimulating lymphatic flow. Skin brushing done concurrently with a gastrointestinal cleaning program improves overall detoxification.

The skin is the largest organ of elimination. It plays a major role in ridding your body of toxins and impurities—potential sources of illness. It is estimated that the skin eliminates over one pound of waste per day. That fact alone should be enough incentive to make you want to brush away those toxins and dead cells. Daily skin brushing is a vital part of an intestinal cleansing program. The skin excretes toxins and poisons present in the body, as do the kidneys and bowels. Dry skin brushing stimulates the sweat glands and increases blood circulation to underlying organs and tissues. Today's sedentary lifestyle, general lack of exercise, and use of antiperspirants keep people from sufficiently perspiring. As a result, toxins and metabolic waste become trapped in the body instead of being released through sweat. Dry skin brushing opens the pores, allows the body to breathe, and enhances healthy organ function.

SKIN BRUSHES

The brush used for lymphatic stimulation should be made of only natural vegetable bristles. Synthetic brushes should be completely *avoided* for this purpose, as they irritate the skin when used dry. A quality skin brush can be purchased through health-food stores and some beauty supply outlets and pharmacies. The brush should be kept dry and not used for bathing. I use a short-handled ergonomically-designed brush. You can also use a long-handled bath brush with a removable head so you can easily control the brushing, only using the long handle for hard-to-reach areas.

The brush and body must be dry. The best time to brush is before taking a bath or shower. Begin by brushing from the outermost points (your hands and feet) toward the center of your body. Pass the brush once over every part of the body surface **except** the face. There should be no back and forth or circular motion, scrubbing, or massaging; one clean sweep is all that's needed. A slight flushing of the skin

Healing Leaky Gut Naturally— *Not* Medicine as Usual

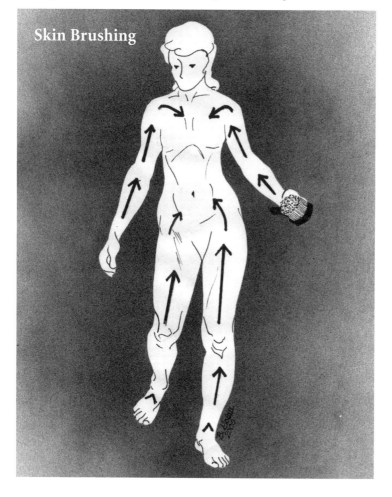

Skin Brushing

is normal due to the increased circulation, but if your skin turns red you're brushing too hard. The total process takes less than one to two minutes. Skin brushing should be performed once or twice per day. It would take thirty minutes or more using a loofah or Turkish towel massage to get similar benefits. When you're finished, take a warm bath or shower. You will feel an invigorating, tingling sensation throughout your body from increased circulation and lymph flow.

It's common for your stools to contain a large amount of lymph mucoid a day or two after starting skin brushing—representing an emptying-out of lymph mucoid backlog present in the lymphatic system. Skin brushing facilitates a lymph-purifying effect.

Colon Health—Waste Management

Colon hydro-therapy saved my life! The detoxifying effects were undeniable when this therapy stopped my frightening symptoms of anaphylactic shock.

Auto-intoxication is the process by which the body literally poisons itself by maintaining a cesspool of decaying matter in the colon. The toxins released by this decay process get into the bloodstream and travel throughout the body. Every cell in the body is affected because toxins weaken the entire system; auto-intoxication and many forms of "incurable diseases" get their start in the colon. An eminent French physician, Bouchard, coined the word "auto-intoxication" and described the various ways diseases may be produced by poisons generated within the body—calling special attention to the intestines, specifically the colon, as a prolific source of poisons. Another source of intestinal poisons is the putrefaction of the protein component of food that fails to undergo absorption.

It is entirely possible for a person to suffer intestinal toxemia without constipation, as in cholera morbus, the diarrheas of infancy, chronic diarrhea, and colitis; it is impossible to have constipation without intestinal auto-intoxication. Intestinal poisoning not manifesting immediate visible effects appear in disorders such as fibromyalgia, chronic fatigue, lupus, arthritis, and other immune system diseases.

My experience proved the effectiveness of two specific methods for reducing the intestinal toxic load of the colon: colon hydro-therapy and enemas.

Colon Hydro-therapy Defined

Colon hydro-therapy is the safe, gentle infusion of water into the colon via the rectum, administered by a certified colon hydro-therapist. No chemicals or drugs are involved and the entire therapy is both relaxing and effective. During therapy the client lies on a custom treatment table in complete comfort. From the hydro-therapy equipment, a small disposable speculum is gently inserted into the rectum, through which warm multi-filtered water passes into the colon.

Modern state-of-the-art colon hydro-therapy units employ multi-stage water purification systems and individual disposables that eliminate possible contamination to the client. A lighted viewing tube allows both the client and therapist to witness contents of elimination. My therapy is performed with what is called a "closed system"—waste is discretely transported into the sewer drain line without offensive odor and without compromising the dignity of the individual and the potential for airborne bacteria. Other systems are available, of which I have minimal personal experience. After each therapy session, the therapist thoroughly cleanses and disinfects the equipment, therapy table, and surrounding areas.

A skilled colon hydro-therapist will use several fills and releases of water to dislodge toxic waste matter adhering to the walls of the colon. The dislodged fecal impactions are then gently washed away through the system's waste-disposal hose. Often a therapist will use a gentle abdominal massage and acupressure during the release process to facilitate elimination.

During the therapy, water temperature and pressure will be monitored by the therapist and can be varied to stimulate muscular contraction (peristalsis) in the colon. This is very important to help a sluggish colon.

Properly administered colon hydro-therapy is not addictive but therapeutic; it encourages the restoration of the colon's natural function by strengthening peristalsis through the reduction of toxic substances that can paralyze rectal muscles.

Each colon hydro-therapy session lasts approximately 45 minutes. Initially, a series of six to twelve separate therapy sessions is generally recommended to begin achieving maximum cleansing benefits. Depending on the toxicity and level of reactions, colon hydro-therapy sessions need to be custom-tailored by a health-care practitioner as part of an overall protocol. Most often they are administered once a week for several weeks. In acute digestive disorders and multiple allergic responses, as in my case, two to three weekly sessions are necessary to control anaphylactic shock and acute reactions until the initial toxic load is reduced, eliminating lodged fecal matter that's been there for weeks, months, and in most cases, years. As healing occurs and reactions subside, the therapy sessions are scheduled further and further apart until a maintenance level is accomplished. The optimum maintenance therapy is two sessions, one week apart, every 3-4 months.

With colon hydro-therapy, the entire large intestine is cleansed and the therapeutic benefits are much greater than those achieved with an enema. Enema cleansing is effective mainly in the rectal area and, due to the body's natural desire to expel, is limited in duration. Often used along with enemas are over-the-counter suppositories. These stimulate expulsion of the contents of the rectum, but contribute to

dehydration, which may exacerbate an already constipated colon.

During typical colon hydro-therapy sessions,
about 25 to 35 gallons of water is transported into
and out of the colon. Using a combination of abdominal massage (if consented by client), reflexology,
breathing instruction, and relaxation techniques, the
colon therapist is often able to promote a great volume of elimination of toxic waste not otherwise possible through individual efforts. *Just one colon hydro-
therapy session may be equivalent to having 20 or 30
regular bowel movements.* Eliminations in subsequent
therapy sessions can be even more substantial as
older, hardened, and impacted feces are dislodged
from the colon walls with the assistance of fiber supplementation and herbal stool softeners.

The therapist will carefully evaluate the client's
progress during each session and will coordinate
therapies with appropriate health-care professionals.

At the onset of therapy, clients with chronic conditions may experience fatigue and a drop in body
temperature. After significant removal of toxins,

Flash-Back

During my illness the only effective method
of eliminating my allergic responses was by professional
colon hydro-therapy with what is called a "closed system"
with regulated water pressure.

most people feel a heightened energy and vitality, and a reduction or elimination of generalized pain, inflammation, and abdominal discomfort.

Colon hydro-therapy provides a proven way to cleanse the colon, thereby increasing the healing process and maintaining optimal health. Remember that maintaining good health is an ongoing process requiring diligence. Your general health probably declined over a period of time; don't expect an immediate return to health. What you can expect is a steady improvement and reduction of symptoms.

Colon hydro-therapy can be most beneficial for restoring good health by:

- clearing the colon of old, hardened, waste material and harmful toxins
- restoring proper pH balance to the body
- stimulating immune functions
- allowing freer passage of nutrients to the blood
- preventing toxic absorption via healthy mucosa
- creating a favorable environment for health-enhancing bacteria and micro-flora

Flash-Forward

I continue to maintain my health, stamina, and endurance by performing colon hydro-therapy every 4-6 weeks. During the months I travel extensively, I keep my toxic load reduced by having therapy as soon as possible when I return, often having it twice a month after long overseas trips.

- strengthening peristaltic activity in the colon and rectum
- promoting a return of normal, regular bowel movements

Millions in this country suffering a myriad of health problems may never consider the source of their problems as a toxic, sluggish colon—not surprising considering conventional methodologies for health disorders and symptoms, and disease management. Using pharmaceuticals and surgery for chronic disorders completely obscures root causes.

Enemas and Colon Cleansing— A Historical Perspective

The invention of this instrument, so essential in maintaining health, belongs to an Italian, Gatenaria, whose name ought to find a modest place together with his countrymen Columbus, Galileo, Gioja, and other eminent and illustrious Italians. Gatenaria was a professor at Pavia, where he died in 1496 after spending several years perfecting his instrument. *The British Medical Journal,* in the late 1800s, describes the invention of the enema apparatus as an epoch in pharmacy as important as the discovery of America in the history of human civilization.

Prior to World War II, it was typical for physicians to recommend enemas for preventive and therapeutic value. Before the drug boom in the 1920s, enemas continued to be widely recommended and written about internationally. In fact, coffee enemas were in the guidebook of medicine, *The Merck Manual of Medical Information*, until 1977. Coffee enemas were used for generations as a way to purge the colon, liver, and gallbladder. (With LGS and MARS the stimulation of coffee can trigger a reaction. I recommend plain, distilled water.) Enema therapy was removed from *The Merck Manual of Medical Information* merely because the space was needed to list all the new drugs on the market—drugs have a higher profit margin than an enema kit!

Whether enemas are the preferred method of colon irrigation, or an adjunct to professional colon hydro-therapy, colon cleansing has a beneficial effect on most ailments, sickness, or disease. The ancient "natural hygiene" philosophy, widely discussed in historical medical books, is that all disease is merely a question of toxicity. Today's reluctance to use colon-cleansing therapies stems from a lack of knowledge of its function and purpose. Our "quick fix" attitudes and demand for symptom-care, rather than health-care, help fuel this reluctance.

You can purchase a reusable enema kit in most drug stores. If you choose to use a disposable hospital bag, you can purchase one at a medical supply store; however, you'll still need the tube and assembly unit. Be sure the water is boiled or distilled. The bag should not be over 18 inches higher than the body, as the enema solution can run into the colon too fast and cause cramping or bloating. Lubricate the tube with pure vitamin E; most lubricants contain ingredients that may cause an irritation or allergic response. The colon hydro-therapist or health-care practitioner can help with specifics on positioning and self-massage techniques to assist in therapy.

Natural Fiber-Cleansing

Everywhere you look, from magazines and newspapers to radio and television, fiber and fiber products are

Flash-Back

Understanding the importance of a colon fiber cleanse, I tried dozens of fiber products and reacted to most of them. Not only did some ingredients precipitate a reaction, they failed to produce regular, sufficient eliminations.

The product I used during my illness was a professional product I was not reactive to. It produced extraordinary results in removing old, putrefied colonic matter. Eventually the company came under new management and my hypersensitive clients and I started to have multiple symptoms not previously experienced because the formula had changed.

To further prove the effectiveness of a fiber colon cleanse, I went so far as to have a medical laboratory perform a pathologic microscopic examination of eliminated rectal tissue. I passed the examined specimen after only two weeks on a fiber colon cleanse. My suspicions were correct, "old necrotic tissue"—likened to a gangrenous condition. With leaky gut, not only was there excessive toxic waste in my colon, it was now circulating throughout my body—literally poisoning me! There's no way of knowing how long this matter sat in my colon becoming more and more toxic. What I do know is that *thanks* to a professionally formulated fiber cleanse product, the gangrenous mass detached and was eliminated.

ıdely talked about and highly advertised. We are literally being bombarded with commercials and advertise-
ments telling us that eating more fiber is not only the
right thing to do, but solves practically all of life's problems. Fiber is essential; however, all fiber and fiber containing complexes are not created equal. Know the facts.

Flash-Forward

I'm happy to report that after diligent
searching for an effective, easily tolerated, all-natural colon
fiber cleanse product, I found ColonSweep®. My clients were
asking for a caplet or capsule—they did not like the flavor or
texture of fiber and botanicals in a powder. ColonSweep is an
easy-to-swallow caplet containing a natural blend of botanicals, essential oils, enzymes, probiotics, multiple fibers, and
alkalizing minerals derived from goat-milk whey. It contains
over 20 proven ingredients to assist the body with cleansing
and detoxification while also supporting liver and gall bladder function with time-tested nutrients. It contains botanicals known to facilitate easy evacuation without dependency—gentle enough for daily use (I take five caplets every
evening) yet successful in facilitating removal of accumulated mucoid plaque (see Resources).

Fiber—Its Functions...

- It improves bowel function. Dietary fiber absorbs
  water in the intestines to provide bulk and soften
  stools, preventing strain.
- It absorbs and eliminates toxins, preventing constipation, hemorrhoids, and diverticulitis.
- It reduces transit time (see explanation in the section "Bowel Transit Time").

- It lowers cholesterol. Vegetable fibers (flax flour, apple fiber powder, psyllium husk and seed powder, and rice bran solubles) can lower the harmful low density lipids (LDL) and raise the valuable protective high density lipids (HDL) cholesterol.
- It reduces the risk of colorectal cancer, a benefit of fiber generally recognized by the American Cancer Society and the Surgeon General of the United States.
- It improves blood-sugar levels. Fiber slows digestion of fats and is believed to reduce the amount of insulin needed.
- It facilitates weight loss. Fiber acts as an appetite suppressant and reduces absorption of fats. It draws water into the intestinal system, creating the sensation of fullness with less caloric intake.

Note: The colon cleansing and fiber-bulking products described in this chapter are what I currently use and recommend.

Uncovering the Past

During a colon cleanse, I always recommend my clients examine their elimination to see what has been packed away and putrefied. This decaying waste material affects other vital organ systems, especially the kidneys and liver, because of circulating toxicity and their burden in attempting to deal with the poisons. As we glance at our bowel elimination, we see the brown color of fecal matter and assume that's all it is. During an effective cleansing program, what you see on the outside is not necessarily what it is. Don't judge elimination by its cover.

At first, the idea of examining your stools may be repugnant. However, the majority of my clients report that after having participated in such an exercise, which takes less than a minute, the results are so apparent (seeing is believing) they actually look forward to watching the progress of ridding their bodies of the accumulated poisonous toxins. We've all had to add some humor to this process, so we coined the phrase "chop sewage," with no disrespect intended to cultures that use chopsticks as utensils.

I started out attempting to find a discrete method of examining my elimination. I found that using a pair of chopsticks worked very well because it allowed me to break apart fecal matter in the commode.

During my initial cleanse, I kept cleansed plastic chopsticks in a small can or receptacle discretely hidden behind the commode in distilled white vinegar to avoid airborne pathogens. Chopsticks made of wood are disposable and preferred. Regardless of what they're made of, they provide an invaluable examination tool. I was eventually gifted an engraved stainless steel pair by a client who had achieved unbelievable results in following my protocols.

While examining your elimination, you may see anything from very large chunks of stringy, black, fibrous mucous alone or covered with parasites, to putrefied slabs of matter that look like raw beefsteak. Keep in mind, the colon fiber cleanse acts as the scouring pad to loosen decayed toxic waste attached to the intestinal walls. With LGS you have additional toxins circulating; consequently, the more accumulated waste removed, the sooner you'll be on the road to recovery.

I recommend examining your eliminations ("chop sewage" method) one week before starting your protocol or cleansing program. This gives you a good comparison before, during, and after the cleansing program. Once you get over the initial idea of examining your stools, you'll be motivated by seeing the progress of your body eliminating substances that are poisoning you, preventing you from achieving optimum health.

An initial period of three months is generally recommended for the cleaning protocol; however, that period can be extended depending upon your specific situation and the advice of your health-care practitioner.

For healthy maintenance, I use and recommend 4-6 caplets each evening anytime after 5 p.m. Cleansing products appear to work best in the evening, preferably 1-2 hours after evening meal, because the body's energy can be used for detoxification rather than everyday functions.

Note: Clients often ask why they should continue to use a vegetable colon fiber cleanse supplement after recovery. It's simple; if you consume at least **two turkey-sized platters of raw vegetables daily**, *you don't need a fiber supplement—5 to 6 caplets of ColonSweep is equivalent to those quantities. I don't know about you, but my jaw aches just thinking about all that chewing, and it's not practical. It's your choice, Naturally.*

Healthy vs. Unhealthy Stool

It's easy to identify a healthy stool. Generally, a medium-brown, well-formed, floating stool with no odor signifies the presence of a healthy, slightly acidic colon pH and the predominance of health-enhancing lacto-bacteria-type intestinal flora. A sinking, dark-colored stool with a bad or foul odor guarantees overgrowth of health-depleting intestinal flora and an alkaline colon.

Many people assume its normal for the stool to have a bad odor. On the contrary, a malodorous stool is perhaps the most significant factor indicating a putrefactive colon—naturally varying from day to day, depending on diet, medications, and other factors. However, you should expect a consistent pattern indicating a healthy stool with slight color variations and no dramatic changes or odor.

Bowel Transit Time

Ideally, food takes 10-12 hours to pass into the colon. Most western (low in fiber) diets have an aver-

I was

Poisoned

by my body...

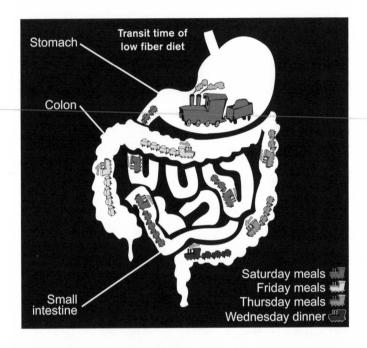

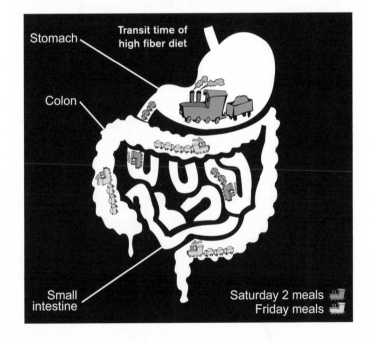

age transit time of 65-100 hours (3 to 10 days, or 9 to 36 meals). This undigested backed-up waste is absorbed into the bloodstream—causing auto-intoxication. Just imagine the volume of 36 digested meals composting in your digestive system! The volume of that much waste could fill a 3-5 gallon container. Remember, if you're consuming three meals a day, and only eliminating once, the remainder is becoming toxic within your body. Is it any wonder we're so toxic?

Food Elimination/Challenge Plan

Charting the Challenger

The consumption reaction connection (CRC) method of testing was one of the first types used for allergy reactive patients. It involves recording what you consume and the allergic responses you experience—assisting in making a connection to offending substances. War on allergens begins with a strategy of attack by first identifying the enemy. It should be executed under the care of a nutritionally aware healthcare practitioner. One of the most helpful suggestions I can share is to record *everything* you consume in a diary. Be careful to read labels identifying *every* ingredient. When an allergic response occurs, knowing specifically what you consumed provides a starting point for the CRC. By doing this exercise you'll be helping yourself and your health-care practitioner identify the causes of your multiple responses.

Food Rotation/Reaction Chart

	(Date) Day 1 Foods Consumed		(Date) Day 2 Foods Consumed
BREAKFAST			
Reaction			
SNACK			
Reaction			
LUNCH			
Reaction			
DINNER			
Reaction			
SNACK			
Reaction			

Food Rotation/Reaction Chart

	(Date) Day 3	Foods Consumed	(Date) Day 4	Foods Consumed
BREAKFAST				
Reaction				
SNACK				
Reaction				
LUNCH				
Reaction				
DINNER				
Reaction				
SNACK				
Reaction				

I was

Poisoned

by my body…

REINTRODUCTION PLAN

When food allergies exist or are suspected, a basic elimination diet is the best approach. In patients such as me, with severe reactions and anaphylactic shock, it is a critical first step. I suggest starting with a modified fast of fresh juices, brown rice, teff, and quinoa, supplemented with a medical-food-quality functional food as a protein-based drink. In my overall initial protocol (previously mentioned) I used functional food therapy as well as a pure organic brown rice protein powder. This product adds only rice protein and no additional nutritional support. However, sometimes it's necessary to start as basic as plain organic rice protein until toxic load is reduced and other proteins and foods can be tolerated. As my tolerance increased, I began alternating between two products that provided protein and supporting nutrients.

At the onset of my allergic reactions and anaphylactic shock, I followed a diet of fresh juice combinations (listed below), brown rice products (including bread, crackers, cereal), and rice milk, with an added rice protein functional food. Any diet regime should be under the guidance of a health-care professional. Do not attempt an elimination diet on your own.

Fresh juices are high in vitamins and especially enzymes. I recommend starting with the following combinations. Remember to start with two or three ingredients so you can chart any adverse reactions. These juice combinations will help the digestive system rest, start the detoxification process, and heal.

- carrot, apple, and ginger
- carrot, celery, and ginger
- carrot, parsley, celery, and ginger
- carrot, apple, parsley, ginger, broccoli stems, or any tolerated green vegetable
- carrot, parsley, beets, apple, celery, ginger

If the concentrated juice causes any stomach distress, dilute the juice with equal parts of pure water.

As you improve and cleanse your liver and colon, fasting on these juices one to two days a week will help speed the healing process of the digestive tract by giving it a rest. Be sure to check with your physician or health-care practitioner before starting any fasting program.

Start with a simple diet of the low-stress foods mentioned above. After two weeks, begin adding other low-allergy ingredients to both your juice and individual foods. For example, if you've been drinking juice made with carrots, apples, and ginger, you can now add beets, parsley, and so forth. If you've been consuming quinoa, add brown rice or an egg (assuming you don't have an allergy to eggs). Make sure to chart how you feel, and look for symptoms of headache, sleeplessness, abdominal bloating, gas, or any other allergic response. When newly introduced foods seem to evoke an allergic response, eliminate them and note how you feel. Don't get discouraged. You will eventually become your own best health detective, and as you reduce the body's overall toxic load and repair the damage, you'll be able to tolerate more and more and finally return to a "normal" diet again. The goal of my consultations and writings is to teach you to take care of your health—no one knows your body better than the one who occupies it.

Flash-Back

At the onset of my illness, it was impossible to focus on a specific diet. The modified fast became my basic safe standby—survival by avoiding allergic responses was foremost. Fresh juices containing carrots and apples, for instance, have natural-occurring sugars that feed *Candida* and parasites. However, the benefits of live enzymes from fresh juice outweigh the sugar factor at this juncture. I did eliminate all other sugar and sugar-containing foods.

At first, I couldn't tolerate any raw vegetables other than a few types that had been juiced. After three weeks of the primary elimination diet and colon hydro-therapy, I was able to add grated carrots and apples, if eaten slowly and in small quantities. Eventually I added any raw vegetable I could consume cooked. Keep in mind that during this time I was dramatically reducing my overall toxic load with colon hydro-therapy, which is why my recovery was accelerated.

The Food Reintroduction Program chart is provided as a guide for slowly reintroducing foods that are best tolerated for individuals experiencing MARS, LGS, and EI—used as part of an overall program of continued detoxification.

As you improve, your body will naturally produce more digestive enzymes; food is better digested, absorption enhanced, and severities of allergic responses decrease. Keep in mind that all people with LGS have *Candida* and/or parasites. Therefore, following a strict diet of eliminating all sugars and sugar-containing foods to starve the *Candida*, along with a cleansing program for parasites, is imperative to overall healing.

Most of my clients with chronic digestive and inflammatory disorders benefit from this elimination/challenge program. Clients who first resisted the program eventually gave it a try after failure with other methods, including medications, which provided no relief. The results were twofold: reduction or elimination of the allergic responses, and help in identifying the offending foods.

Leaky Gut—Food Reintroduction Program

Consume all foods as tolerated.

VEGETABLES
Beets & Tops
Broccoli
Carrot
Celery
Chard
Chives
Garlic
Green Peas
Leeks
Onions/Scallions
Pumpkin
Snow Peas
Spaghetti Squash
Spinach
String Beans
Summer Squash
Sweet Potatoes
Swiss Chard
Wheatgrass Juice
Winter Squash
Yams
Zucchini

MEAT & EGGS
Cornish Hen
Deep Cold Water Fish
Organic Chicken
Organic Eggs
Organic Turkey

FATS, OILS & NUTS
Avocado
Finely Ground Almonds
Ghee
Macadamia Nut Oil
Olive Oil
Organic Real Butter
Pumpkin Seed Oil
Safflower Oil
Sesame Seed Oil
Sunflower Oil

STARCH/GRAINS
Brown Basmati Rice
Brown Rice Long Grain
Brown Rice Bread
Brown Rice Cakes
Brown Rice Chips
Brown Rice Crackers
Cream of Rice
Quinoa
Quinoa Flake Cereal
Rice Cereal
Rice Pancakes
Rice Pasta
Tapioca
Teff

CHEESE & DAIRY
Almond Cheese
Goat Milk Products
Rice Cheese
Sheep Milk Products

HERBS/SPICES
Apple Mint
Borage
Basil
Bay leaf
Cilantro
Coriander
Dill
Ginger
Lavender
Mint
Parsley
Rosemary
Saffron
Sage
Tarragon
Thyme
Turmeric

SOUPS
Homemade Vegetarian
Vegetable-based Broths
Chicken Broth

FRUIT
Apples & Applesauce
Grapes (in moderation)
Guava (in moderation)
Kiwi
Mango
Melons (well washed)
Organic Applesauce
   (glass container)
Organic Plum
   Sauce (glass container)
Papaya
Plum Sauce
Unsweetened
   Applesauce (glass
   container)
Watermelon
Berries (seedless,
   puree, or jelly)

BEVERAGES
Almond Milk
Berry Juice
   (no seeds or sugar)
Chamomile Tea
Fennel Tea
Ginger Tea
Hazelnut Milk
Non-citrus herb teas
Rice Carob Milk
Rice Milk
Slippery Elm Tea
Unsweetened fruit juice
Unsweetened vegetable
   juice (all juices should
   be bottled)
Teeccino® Herbal Coffee

With this dietary plan you rotate foods—every day for five days you consume only certain vegetables, grains, fruits, and sources of protein, as tolerated. The following foods are the largest contributors of food allergies, and should be avoided:

- Wheat
- Dairy (unless made from goat or sheep milk—usually tolerated by sensitive individuals)
- Eggs
- Yeast
- Peanuts
- Gluten-containing foods
- Corn

After five days, the cycle begins again, so what you eat on Day One you can eat again on Day Six, and what you eat on Day Two you can repeat on Day Seven. This system allows a full four days without repeating a food.

A Little is Safe—Repetition CAN Trigger Allergic Responses

By rotating foods you're calling to work only certain enzymes on that day, allowing other systems the opportunity to recover. Also, like the elimination diet, the rotation dietary plan makes it easy for you to identify which foods are causing problems. It is important to eat a variety of foods; however, those of us with LGS can't always include all food groups at first. After you start detoxifying and healing, you'll be able to regain tolerance to most previously reactive foods.

Once you identify and eliminate a food you're responsive to for 4-6 weeks or longer, you can again possibly reintroduce it. Be cautious and include only small quantities on a rotated schedule—reducing the risk your body will again be reactive to it.

It is very important to maintain rotation for **everything** you consume, including protein drinks and functional foods. Most supplements don't have to be rotated, but if you can tolerate one and then react, rotate.

These recommendations are primary tools, not cast in concrete; listen to your body!

Flash-Back

I was starving for protein and, as a result of that, lost my muscle tone. I was so excited when a client brought me my first batch of organic, creamy, smooth, home-made goat cheese that I ate several tablespoons a day for several days. On the seventh day, my throat closed and I had a full-blown allergic response again.

The significance of the seventh day should have been my first clue. I didn't allow my digestive system to rest from the newly introduced food, so my body stopped me in my tracks. I was so discouraged. My body not only needed the animal protein, it craved it! After two weeks of abstinence, I reintroduced the same type of cheese, with no problems. I then added this delicacy to my rotational diet.

The following books are excellent resources for allergy and rotational diets. They are helpful as you introduce new and unusual foods and combinations.

- *5 Years Without Food—The Food Allergy Survival Guide*, Nicolette Dumke, Adapt Books 1998.
- *If This is Tuesday, It Must Be Chicken*, Natalie Golos and Frances Golos Golbitz, Keats Publishing 1983.
- *Allergy & Candida Cooking Made Easy*, Sondra Lewis, Canary Connect Publications 1996.
- *Organic Gourmet*, Leslie Cerier, Station Hill Openings-Barrytown, Ltd. 1996.

General Dietary Life-Style Changes

Water, Water, Water

Our bodies are approximately 70 percent water. Its water supply is responsible for running digestion, absorption, circulation, and elimination processes. Replacing the water continually lost through sweat and elimination is essential. Additionally, if you do not consume enough water during a cleansing and detoxifying routine, you endanger tissue health because concentrated toxins are being eliminated from your cells and colon and must be flushed. Water is vital. Dehydration can have such damaging effects that lack of water can lead to death. The body can survive without food for approximately four to six weeks; without water it can only exist for about five days.

I find it very helpful to drink water out of a bottle

with a built-in straw. I have a 32-ounce sipper bottle in every location: car, office, and home. Somehow the sipping action encourages larger quantity with less effort. Most plastics are not healthy for anyone, especially if you have chemical sensitivities. Use caution and drink out of glass or paper and use glass or paper straws. My bottles are made of a material that does not leach contaminants—unfortunately they are no longer made.

Dr. Batmanghelidj, author of *Your Body's Many Cries for Water*, recommends drinking *half of your body weight in ounces*. For example, if you weigh 160 pounds, you need to consume 80 ounces of water each day (equal to 10 cups). A 200-pound individual needs to drink 100 ounces of water each day (equal to $12^1/2$ cups).

Clients report that, although challenging at first, within two weeks of drinking through a straw their body craves more water. Drinking pure water allows your body to flush toxins without having to mobilize the digestive system. Caffeine-free tea, hot or cold, counts for part of your daily intake. However, be careful with some herbal teas containing ingredients with stimulating effects; they make your body systems work instead of resting and restoring. Drinking water with fresh lemon is beneficial for most people; however, with LGS, citrus can cause disturbing responses and inflammation. It's best to get into a routine of just plain, pure, water, water, water.

There are 1,500,000,000 pounds of pesticides used in the United States each year on agricultural food products alone. This equates to nearly five pounds of poisonous sprays for each person. Approximately 45,000 different agricultural chemicals are used, 150 of these regularly appear as residue in food, with over two dozen of them at toxic levels.

IF THE BUGS WON'T EAT THEM, WHY SHOULD WE?

Why subject yourself and your family to the effects of these chemicals, when you can purchase or grow organic foods? Yes, it takes some planning, but don't wait until your allergic responses reach the level of anaphylactic shock or cancer before you change your choice of food. Make sure produce is labeled "Certified Organically Grown." This is the best assurance the food

Flash-Back

Every time I consumed non-organic food, I reacted within 12-15 minutes. When consuming the same certified organic food, I experienced no reaction. During my illness, my entire diet consisted of only organic foods.

Flash-Forward

Added awareness of the health importance of organic foods has created a high demand and now most grocers are filling their shelves with organics.

is truly organic—anything less is questionable. Organic foods bring us health, not disease. They generally cost more than conventionally grown food, but as powerfully stated by Leslie Cerier, author of *The Organic Gourmet*, organic foods are "the cheapest health insurance around for you, your family, and the environment."

Our bodies were not engineered to process synthetic substances.

Always wash all produce with either a store-bought vegetable wash to remove residue of chemicals or make your own solution. Here are two formulas:

1. *Use 15 drops of liquid grape seed extract to a quart of water. Stir vigorously; the serum is very oily. Rinse the food for about 2-4 minutes to remove oily pesticides on fruits and veggies.

2. *Use 2 TB. hydrogen peroxide to one quart of water. Soak vegetables or fruit for 2-4 minutes.

Note: Scrub vegetables and fruit vigorously with a vegetable brush and rinse well before soaking in a cleansing solution such as those above.

SMALLER, MORE FREQUENT MEALS

For a victim of severe allergic responses with a toxic colon, it is essential to nourish the body frequently and in small portions. This way of eating is not unlike a routine diabetic diet, small amounts of food every $1^1/2$ to $2^1/2$ hours. It's important to keep the body nourished and blood-sugar levels neutral, while not overworking the digestive system.

Flash-Forward

As mentioned earlier in this book, it is difficult, if not impossible, for me to consume only certified organic food when away from home. Living by the 80/20 rule has allowed me to travel and eat in four or five star restaurants with no allergic responses—I'm teased by friends and colleagues that I'm an expensive, but healthy, date. Better restaurants make their food from scratch, providing the opportunity for me to ask questions about specific ingredients that I must avoid (preservatives, additives, flavor enhancers and nightshades). The 80/20 rule cannot apply, however, until the body has been detoxified and the gut repaired. In addition, keep in mind that ongoing detoxification and environmental protocols must be maintained such as colon fiber supplements, periodic colon cleansing and stimulation of the lymphatic system (rebounding, skin brushing, lymphatic massage) and an indoor environment as free of toxic substances as possible.

The "Whey" to Supplement Minerals

We Are Electrical Creatures

Minerals comprise the body's electrical transmission system, providing commands (responses) to every cell, and transmission of brain signals through body fluids. Intestinal disorders, particularly LGS, cause a deficiency of minerals.

There are two groups of minerals, macro-minerals (bulk) and micro-minerals (trace).

- **Macro-minerals** include calcium, magnesium, sodium, potassium, and phosphorus. For proper electrical transmission, the body needs these minerals in larger amounts than trace minerals. Muscle cramping and pain are common symptoms in inflammatory and intestinal disorders—symptoms are usually the result of mineral depletion or imbalance. Deficiency can also occur as a result of excessive consumption of water, dietary salt, some prescription drugs, and colon irrigation.

- **Micro-minerals** include zinc, iron, copper, manganese, chromium, selenium, and iodine. These minerals are needed in only minute quantities; however, they are critical for balanced health and healing.

Minerals are stored primarily in the body's bone and muscle tissue. The absorbed mineral must be carried by the blood to the cells and then absorbed by the cell membrane to be utilized. When the mineral enters the body through the intestinal lining, it competes with other minerals for absorption; therefore, minerals should always be taken in balanced proportions.

EXAMPLES OF MINERAL IMBALANCES

Excessive consumption of:	*Causes depletion of:*
• Zinc	• Copper and iron
• Calcium	• Magnesium and zinc
• Copper	• Zinc
• Phosphorus	• Calcium

Much of what we consume in modern diets is stripped of nutrients from chemical farming, food processing, synthetic food additives and preservatives, and soil that is depleted of minerals. No wonder our health and quality of life is slowly eroding from consuming foods meant to sustain it!

Minerals are the spark-plugs of life, necessary for every function—without them there is no life. They are the body's electrical transmitters, igniting electrical stimuli to every cell.

In my experience, the most effective natural mineral/electrolyte replacement is from goat-milk whey. It is processed at low temperatures to retain nutritional integrity, and contains more than 20 naturally-occurring minerals as a highly complex whole food. Because of its high sodium, potassium, and calcium content, mineral whey has an alkaline reaction, creating a healthy pH for repair and health maintenance.

The most plentiful mineral ingredients in mineral whey are the electrolytes. These electrolytes make up the electrically charged ions that help regulate water balance, acid-alkaline balance, osmotic pressure, nerve impulse conduction, muscle contraction and transport into and out of the cells.

The typical analysis of whey confirms its nutritional benefits: high in natural amino acids and minerals, and containing some vitamins. The soluble protein lactoglobulins in whey are identical to serum globulin in human blood and contain antibodies that help strengthen immune functions. The major soluble proteins in whey are beta-lactoglobulin, immunoglobulin, alpha-lactalbumin, and serum albumin. These amino acids are rated higher in bio-availability than those in eggs, according to the World Health Organization. Additionally, research shows whey protein is superior to soy, rice, wheat, and beef for quality overall bio-availability. Colon function thrives when provided with mineral whey because natural, whole, sweet whey is the ideal food to promote the growth of healthy colon flora.

The product I use for mineral replacement and supplementation is Capra Mineral Whey™. It is a mineral-rich, golden brown, dry natural food powder from dehydrated natural goat-milk whey. This form of whole food has shown superior reduction or elimination of symptoms, with a greater absorption factor than tablets or capsules from other sources.

Mineral whey provides excellent mineral supplementation for digestive disorders and particularly after diarrhea, enemas, and colon therapy, when minerals are lost along with toxic debris. It can be taken in water or juice, sprinkled onto hot or cold cereal, mixed with any food where sweetening is appropriate, or as a "hot toddy" in boiling water. The powder is naturally very sweet and tasty. It does not mix well in cool water unless added to a protein shake and blended as I do.

"My Whey"

203

Healing Leaky
Gut Naturally—
Not Medicine
as Usual

"Whey to go!" It's amazing how quickly those "charley horses" went trotting off somewhere else, rather than over my legs.

Goat-milk mineral whey powder eliminated my muscle spasms and aches within three days of initial consumption. I took two tablespoons in a small amount of water or juice three times daily. After several months, I reduced the amount to two tablespoons, once daily. If muscle spasms reoccur, I increase the amount for a few days until symptoms are eliminated. When spasms reoccur after disappearing, it is important to determine what changed in the daily routine to cause depletion of minerals. Possible causes are excessive sweating, frequent colon irrigation (more than once a week), excessive intake of carbonated drinks or coffee, and diarrhea.

Flash-Back

I used a colloidal organic liquid mineral supplementation before developing leaky gut. Afterward, I couldn't take it without experiencing an allergic response. Researching and comparing ingredients, I concluded most colloidal mineral combinations contained citric acid or additional ingredients, not well tolerated by a compromised gut, including mine.

Fiber *decreases* absorption of minerals, so take supplemental fiber or bulking supplements at different times. It is best, but not always possible, to wait

4-6 hours between mineral supplementation and fiber products. For example, take a fiber supplement in the evening and mineral supplementation in the morning and during the day.

Nutritional Support and Vitamin Supplementation

Proteins—A Quick Reference

The foundation of complete health is formed by the presence of protein and its billions of biochemical activities.

This guide is provided as a quick-reference to assist you in understanding not only the importance of protein, but also the differences between complete and incomplete proteins.

Protein is essential to life—your health, stamina, quality of life and performance depend on it and the body's ability to easily and effectively digest and utilize it.

IMPORTANCE OF PROTEIN

- makes up 90 percent of dry blood weight, 80 percent of muscles, and 70 percent of skin
- provides building blocks for connective tissue
- acts as a primary constituent of enzymes, hormones, and antibodies
- encompasses vital chemicals like immunoglobulins
- forms the foundation of muscles, skin, bones, hair, heart, teeth, blood, brains, and billions of

biochemical activities performed within our bodies every minute of the day.

MANIFESTATIONS OF PROTEIN DEFICIENCY

- chronic fatigue
- muscle and connective tissue disorders (fibromyalgia, myalgic fibromyositis, myofascial pain syndromes, muscle fatigue, spasms)
- deteriorating and/or blurred vision
- depression
- slow wound healing
- decreased resistance to infection
- grayish complexion
- hair loss
- interruption or stoppage of female menstruation
- fragile, splitting and slow-growing fingernails
- lack of physical endurance (especially for exercise)

TYPES OF PROTEIN

Incomplete Protein
- derived from vegetable sources
- low in essential amino acids even when consumed in high amounts

Complete Protein
- derived from animal sources—the only complete protein
- contains all essential amino acids

Whey Protein
- Researchers confirm that, when whey protein is consumed by itself, it produces too rapid an absorption of amino acids, utilizing them strictly for energy production instead of tissue building as well.

Goat-milk Protein
- It is easier to digest and absorb because of its smaller protein molecules—most like human milk. It is better tolerated by those highly allergic or reactive to cow's milk and those with compromised/damaged digestive systems.

Perfect Balanced Protein®
- derived from a balanced blend of goat-milk and goat-milk whey proteins
- provides a complete compliment of essential body-building blocks, including glutamine
- provides a healthy ratio of potassium to sodium— just the way nature intended, as found in whole milk
- is lacto-fermented, containing super strains of naturally-occurring probiotics (health-enhancing bacteria)
- is fermented by lactic acid bacteria, creating biologically active lactic acid that supports energy production and fat-burning
- establishes a proper pH balance within the G.I. tract and body tissues

Flash-Forward

The perfect balanced goat-milk protein I referred to earlier in this book and the one I use in my daily shakes is Caprotein™. Goat-milk and products derived from it provided protein nutrition to rebuild my health, restore my muscle tone, and assisted the repair of my digestive system—now they facilitate health maintenance.

In my 30+ years of nutrition and detoxification counseling, the health benefits of goat-milk never cease to amaze me. It is, after all, the most widely consumed milk in the world, and for good reason, credited for supporting stamina and longevity by the healthiest and longest living people. It is the perfect choice for those who are striving to repair their digestive system, as well as for those of us who have recovered and live busy, demanding lives. It's nutritious, tasty, and essentially nature's "original fast-food" (see Resources).

Glutamine—Essential for Intestinal Repair

Glutamine is an amino acid derived from the fermentation process of grain and then purified so as to eliminate any potential allergic responses. Glutamine is a preferred fuel for cells that make up your gastrointestinal tract, as well as your immune system—primarily energy fuel for the small intestine.

Glutamine is a non-essential amino acid, meaning that in a healthy person it is normally produced at sufficient rates to adequately supply glutamine-consuming tissues. Of all the amino acids incorporated into protein, *glutamine is the most abundant in the human body.*

In the patient with nutritional depletion, common with food allergies, LGS, and intestinal disorders, decreased muscle tissue and changes in intermediary metabolism lead to diminished glutamine production. This depletion results in decreased availability and uptake of plasma glutamine concentration in the gut.

Laboratory studies show that parts of the immune system (especially liver and spleen) switch from release of glutamine to consumption of glutamine after a trauma. The hypothesis is that in a depleted state, such as loss of muscle mass, the capacity to produce sufficient glutamine for the immune system diminishes—the consequence is deterioration of the gut mucosal barrier.

The digestive tract uses glutamine not only as a fuel source, but also for healing stomach ulcers, irritable bowel, ulcerative bowel diseases, and LGS. It is additionally used to sooth the digestive tract in celiac patients and is the most used anti-ulcer nutrient in Asia. Basically, glutamine helps heal the leaky cells and is a fuel source that facilitates healing of the entire digestive tract; supplementing the body's natural supply of glutamine short-circuits the body's need to borrow from its own muscle tissue. Lost muscle tone is especially evident in inflammatory disorders such as fibromyalgia.

Glutamine also helps maintain healthy glutathione (GSH) levels. Glutathione is considered by many experts to be the most important antioxidant produced by the body.

The goal of glutamine supplementation is to diminish damage to your GI tract, decrease symptoms, and enhance the antioxidant and immune response systems. As a bonus, glutamine supports healthy brain function and is considered "brain fuel." Anyone suffering the consequences of LGS, MARS/EI, and digestive disorders appreciates any brain fuel we can get!

Supplementation with pure glutamine is essential and is included in BioInflammatory Plus, one of the functional food formulas described at the beginning of this chapter.

Ginger—A Natural Digestive Aid

Ginger root (*Zingiber officinale*) is an ancient herb used extensively for thousands of years in Chinese, Ayurvedic, and Western healing modalities. It's a flavorful condiment, a stimulating and warming tea, or tasty raw in fresh juices. Ginger is especially beneficial in cases of exhaustion from chronic disease because it strengthens the entire body. Cleansing heals but also puts stress on the digestive system. Ginger assists neutralization of stress from detoxification. Because of its anti-inflammatory properties, ginger is effective in pain management, reduction of gas/bloating, indigestion, and nausea. Studies show ginger is at least as effective as prescription drugs for general nausea and motion sickness, without the potential side-effects. I recommend using ginger in cooking, stir-fry, and particularly in fresh juice (see recipes in Food Elimination/Challenge Reintroduction Plan).

Ginger—Its Health Benefits

- cleanses the colon, stomach, small intestine, circulatory system, and liver
- stimulates circulation
- reduces spasms
- eases muscle cramps
- increases bile secretion
- antioxidant protection for the liver
- antibacterial properties
- anti-parasitic properties
- protects the heart by lowering cholesterol and inhibiting platelet aggregation
- normalizes bowel function
- restores colon tone
- assists digestion
- eliminates/reduces nausea

Aloe Vera Juice—Nature's Tissue Repair and Anti-inflammatory

As far back as I remember, I was told about the miraculous benefits of the aloe vera plant. Raised by my paternal grandmother, a natural herbalist, it was impossible for me to avoid learning about herbs. I remember aloe vera growing on our patio in Southern California. Every time someone had a skin burn or digestive heartburn grandma ran out to pluck a leaf. As a child, I accepted most of this information as "old wives' tales" only to find out later what has been proven for centuries: your house isn't complete if aloe vera isn't growing in your patio or home.

Years later, scientific research confirms the boundless powers of aloe vera doing exactly what the "old wives tales" proclaimed:

- eases pain and heals wounds caused by searing, scalding, sunburn, radiation, and other types of burns
- heals skin ulcerations, relieves dermatitis, seborrhea, and acne
- proven effective against peptic and oral ulcers
- cleanses infections and retards fungus growth
- provides superior, totally natural cosmetic benefits
- encapsulated herbal form produces a gentle natural laxative effect
- unequaled in soothing and healing the entire digestive tract from heart burn, gastroesophageal reflux disease (GERD) and intestinal inflammation

These documented matters of record regarding use of aloe vera are a testament to history repeating itself. The results are published in some of the most prestigious scientific journals and textbooks of medical literature. The aloe plant was used by ancient civilizations and given the common name of Curacao or Barbados Aloe—suggesting a New World origin. However, aloe vera is native to the Mediterranean region of southern Europe and North Africa. Using the juice of the aloe

Flash-Forward

Even my clients who insisted they were allergic to aloe juice were amazed they didn't react to the one I recommend—I had already been the guinea pig and the health detective, and experienced amazing improvement. I now take one ounce of distilled aloe vera juice once a day for maintenance, many times adding it to my protein drink. I always carry a 2-ounce bottle for those times when I eat out and the food produces heartburn, for whatever reason. It eliminates my distress within fifteen minutes and is especially convenient because it doesn't require refrigeration.

plant as a cathartic (laxative) goes back to the early days of Greece and Rome. The plant was introduced into the Caribbean in the seventeenth century to be cultivated for its juice, which was then evaporated and exported back to Europe as a remedy for constipation.

Aloe vera is a member of the lily family, but it does not resemble its distant cousin. Aloe vera is a perennial succulent that is drought-resistant. The outside skin of the leaf is smooth, fairly thick, with a rubbery texture. Right below the outside layer are the cells that secrete the juice used to make aloe products. The inner chamber is made up of the clear gel, or pulp, resembling slightly melted lemon Jell-O®. The pulp is believed by the Russians to contain wound-healing agents called "biogenic stimulators."

You can purchase aloe vera juice in health-food stores and pharmacies but you must be aware of the differences. The only one that my clients and I have been able to consume without an allergic response is one that is fractionally distilled, available from health-care professionals, called Professional's Care®. There is a mild laxative element with aloe in capsules, but *not with the juice*. It is my belief that allergic responses occur to other forms of aloe juice because they either have additives or coloring or form microscopic bacteria, especially if not properly refrigerated after opening. The one I use and recommend looks, tastes, and feels like water—distillation makes it appear like water. The distillation process removes potential allergens and the bitter taste. Additionally, Professional's Care contains no preservatives or additives and is completely aloin free.

The juice protects the mucous membranes and, therefore, has a healing and soothing effect on the entire digestive tract. In constipation or diarrhea, it will assist in returning the stools to normal. In addition, I find aloe vera juice to be effective for food allergies and to protect the digestive system when it's necessary to take medications. I routinely took two ounces (a jigger full) of aloe vera juice three times a day and the effects were very calming to an angry stomach or gut.

Candida—Fighting Your Fungus

It's been scientifically reported that antibiotics change the balance of intestinal micro-flora—they *kill both health-enhancing and health-depleting bacteria* throughout the body, specifically in the digestive system. This creates the perfect condition for bacteria, parasites, viruses, and yeasts that are resistant to antibiotics. In a healthy intestinal tract, these harmful bacteria may be present in small numbers without any adverse responses or symptoms. However, once overgrowth occurs, they produce waste material that becomes poisonous chemicals to body cells. *Candida albicans* (yeast) is nothing new to the medical profession. Ralph Golan, M.D. clearly stated, "At one extreme, it can cause skin rashes or vaginal infections (*mucocutaneous candidiasis*). At the other extreme, in individuals whose immune systems are severely compromised, yeast can invade the bloodstream (candidemia) and cause death." Your present LGS, and the accompanying *Candida*, may not yet have reached life-threatening proportions, but do present a major roadblock to healing.

In real estate it's been said that a piece of property is only as good as its location, location, location. In healing the LGS, managing and eliminating *Candida* is essential and that effectiveness depends primarily on diet, diet, diet. The challenge for the LGS patient is that a typical *Candida* diet cannot be strictly followed due to the allergic responses, gut consequences, and the resulting generalized malnutrition. Therefore, the following guidelines are provided in general terms to assist you in avoiding foods that directly contribute to yeast growth. The guidelines do not apply during the acute time of healing the LGS, unless your tolerance for foods is better than mine was.

When the following guidelines are strictly adhered to for approximately 12 weeks, the body will suffocate or starve the yeast fungus. In some cases, there is an initial worsening of symptoms as the yeast die off (Herxheimer reaction) and the associated toxins circulate. The yeast organism eats first, leaving you with the leftovers—toxic by-products of their digestion and actual die-off. Colon cleansing at this phase of detoxification is essential. After two to four weeks (be sure to check with your health-care practitioner), you should feel a relief of symptoms and renewed physical and emotional energy. Eliminating overgrowth of *Candida* requires a life-long commitment to eliminating sugars and sugar-forming foods. Once the gut is healed and overgrowth eliminated, the occasional sweet treat can generally be tolerated.

What to Avoid

- *Sugar and sugar-containing foods*—Sugar is sugar, whether it's refined or unrefined, such as turbinado, dried cane juice, raw sugar, honey, maple syrup, or molasses. Be aware, read labels—sugar comes in many disguises. *Candida* multiplies at an alarming rate in a sugary environment. Fruit, including that in fresh juices, should be limited to a daily maximum of one serving. Fruits contain mostly sugar, so limit yourself to a half piece of fruit for one serving or as many small fruits as will fit in the palm of your hand.

One whole apple or half an apple and a small bunch of grapes would constitute your total daily allotment.

- *Artificial Sweeteners**—NutraSweet® and Equal® (aspartame) have been known to cause severe allergic responses, both physically and psychologically, known as neurotoxins.
- *Cheese and dairy*—Avoid all processed and aged cheeses. Organic fresh goat and sheep cheese is acceptable in moderate amounts. Milk and milk

Flash-Forward

HEALTHY SUGAR ALTERNATIVE

I use and recommend a natural herbal sweetener named SweetLife®, made from the Chinese plant Lo Han. It is 300 times sweeter than sugar and is combined with the carrier fructose in order to reduce the potency of its flavor. The added fructose does not significantly affect blood sugar levels or *Candida* and is approved by the Diabetes Resource Center as safe for diabetics.

Fructose is a low glycemic sugar that naturally occurs in fruit and berries. It is slowly absorbed in the small intestine and mainly metabolized in the liver. Compared to sucrose (table sugar) containing a glycemic index of 92, fructose has a glycemic index of 32.

Each serving of SweetLife contains less than one gram of sugar (from fructose). An average size Granny Smith apple contains 25 grams. It would take 25 servings of SweetLife to equal the sugar content of one Granny Smith apple. It contains no calories and less than one gram of sugar and dietary fiber.

It's great for baking and cooking and it's what I add to my protein shakes each day. The powder is available in a shaker bottle or boxed in individual serving packets (see Resources).

products are simple carbohydrates, which feed yeast.

- *Yeast-containing foods*—Avoid breads and pastries that are yeast-leavened.

Flash-Forward

HEALTHY COFFEE ALTERNATIVE

I am a coffee connoisseur; I like the aroma and flavor. After researching the health-depleting effects of caffeine and experiencing allergic responses, I set out on a mission to locate a product that would satisfy the coffee lover in me while supporting my health.

A colleague introduced me to a naturally caffeine-free herbal coffee named Teeccino® (tea-chee-no). I was pleasantly surprised that it contained all the qualities I enjoy in coffee, without caffeine—its ingredients are actually health-enhancing.

Teeccino is blended from natural ingredients that are roasted and ground to brew and taste just like coffee, without the caffeine and acidity.

Take a look at the health benefits of Teeccino; they'll surprise you and your palette.

- naturally caffeine-free—no processing or chemical residues
- high in heart-healthy potassium
- provides a natural energy boost—from nutrients, not stimulants
- is alkaline—helps reduce acidity and restore alkaline (pH) balance
- is rich in inulin—a soluble fiber in chicory root; helps improve digestion and elimination and increases the absorption of calcium and minerals

It comes in a variety of flavors; my favorite is mocha! For complete details about the health-benefits of Teeccino, and to learn why decaf is not a healthy substitute for coffee, refer to articles and information on my website at www.gloriagilbere.com.

- *Alcoholic beverages*—Avoid beer and wine fermented and/or brewed with yeast.
- *Gluten-containing grains*—Avoid especially wheat, oats, rye, and barley.
- *Fungi and moldy foods*—Avoid citric acid, truffles, morels, mushrooms, and tempeh—a white cultured mold closely related to the mushroom.
- *Vinegar-containing foods*—Avoid mustard, ketchup, steak sauces, barbecue sauces, green olives, horseradish, mayonnaise, pickles, and most store-bought salad dressings.
- *Fermented products*—Avoid root beer, cider, soy sauce, miso, and tamari. A healthy substitute is Braggs Amino Acids®, a naturally fermented soy product and a good replacement for traditional soy sauce (available at most health food stores).
- *Dried or canned fruits*—Dried fruits become a highly concentrated sugar and can collect mold. Canned fruit is processed, and therefore, should be avoided when possible.
- *Caffeine-containing products*—Avoid coffee, tea, chocolate, and other foods containing caffeine. Substituting carob for chocolate is acceptable. Carob-flavored rice milk is a delicious substitute for chocolate milk (see Flash-Forward page 217).

Garlic—Its Health Benefits

In 1858, Louis Pasteur first proved garlic to be a natural antibiotic. His research demonstrated the ability of garlic to kill bacteria in laboratory culture dishes.

Dr. Benjamin Lau, famed immunologist, conducted experiments testing the ability of various powerful drugs to stop the growth of bacteria and fungi. His findings proved garlic extract stopped the growth of those cultures even more effectively than the drugs being used for the same purpose. His research confirmed garlic to be an effective, broad-spectrum antibiotic and anti-fungal.

His research also concluded that garlic worked particularly on the mold that causes *Candida albicans,* acting on the lipid layer of the cell membrane. It interfers with lipid synthesis and with the yeast organism's ability to take up oxygen. In other words, garlic causes these microbes to lose their membrane, the lining of their structure—depriving them of the ability to breathe. Studies confirmed what the Chinese have known for centuries: garlic inhibits viral multiplication.

In winning the battle with *Candida*, diet control is major; however, I also recommend additional supplements that assist in killing yeast faster, after detoxification processes are started to reduce the existing toxic load. Garlic is one natural supplement that kills yeast overgrowth without the side-effects of drugs. In LGS-type syndromes, and the accompanying *Candida*, the addition of supplemental garlic speeds recovery, minimizing infection. Start slowly by adding a small fresh piece to your food or fresh juice, then take a garlic supplement to avoid symptoms of die-off.

According to research conducted in the Department of Microbiology at the University of Oklahoma, garlic juice is as effective as the anti-fungal drugs Amphotericin® and Nystatin®. Researchers confirm the benefits of garlic. Next came the challenge of producing socially acceptable garlic, without the taste and odor.

Garlic—Socially Acceptable Supplementation

The beneficial constituent of garlic is the alliin—the higher the alliin count, the greater the benefit. Scientific studies presented at the World Garlic Conference (1990) stated categorically that cooked garlic and garlic extract in liquid or powdered form have the same properties as raw garlic.

Many brands of garlic are available. Manufacturers of garlic capsules and tablets have successfully found a way of maintaining the alliin benefits without the taste and odor. You will, at times, detect the fragrance of garlic when opening a bottle in supplemental form. However, this doesn't mean you will taste or

Flash-Forward

I do not have allergic responses to garlic.
I take a professional brand that contains 700 mg. per capsule and I take one a day unless my sugar intake has been higher, then I increase it to two, always with food.

smell like garlic. If you use a brand that does stimulate body odor, change brand. The difference in body chemistry accounts for various responses to different brands.

To receive long-term benefits, it's important for garlic to be supplemented daily, not as a random "quick fix." However, just as important as consistency is the correct amount of supplementation. Check with your health-care practitioner before starting supplementation. In LGS and digestive disorders, excessive supplemental garlic may cause destruction of the body's beneficial bacteria within the digestive tract. In rare cases, toxicity and swelling of the liver can occur if **raw** garlic is consumed in excessive amounts.

Liver Detoxification and Support

The liver is the organ that bears the burden of faulty digestion and LGS. In my case, the liver symptoms included jaundice skin, yellowish color to whites of eyes, chronic swelling under right breast, and acute sharp pains. The following therapies and supportive supplements were critical in my healing process.

Note: It's important to cleanse the colon before embarking on a liver detoxification program. Colon cleansing reduces the amount of waste and toxins circulated through the liver, allowing the liver to start the repair processes. Once a disease has been established as chronic, you must suspect suppressed liver detoxification. Although at times difficult to measure, liver toxi-

city adds up to the total amount of toxins and its ability to eliminate them. Ultimately, liver health predicts the overall health of the individual.

Homeopathic Support

A special clinical homeopathic blend provided me with natural support during and after the detoxification process. It is supplied in liquid form—several

Flash-Back

After developing LGS, for weeks I couldn't tolerate any form of supplemental support for the liver, except the homeopathic remedy mentioned above. When the liver became swollen, I took one drop daily in eight ounces of water and slowly sipped throughout the day to avoid "dumping" of toxins too quickly and causing more discomfort.

Flash-Forward

The maximum dose of RxDrainer is six drops daily at bedtime. Because of my extreme liver dysfunction from prescription medications for pain and inflammation, it took me one year after my accident to be able to slowly work up to six drops, which I continue to take daily to maintain my health.

I have clients that are so hypersensitive they place one drop in 16-32 ounces of water daily, take one sip, and discard what remains. As their body's toxic load is reduced by overall detoxification protocols, they slowly decrease the amount of water and eventually tolerate one drop directly under the tongue. If increasing the amount of homeopathic causes backache in the kidney region or liver pain, it's a sign the level of toxins in the liver and kidneys have exceeded the organs' capacity to neutralize and purge them.

drops taken sublingually (under the tongue) as recommended by your health-care practitioner. More often than not with LGS and chronic disorders, the homeopathic remedy provides gentle support without causing rapid detoxification and triggering a response in the liver or kidneys. The complex I use is called "RxDrainer®"—a blend of homeopathic ingredients to stimulate liver, kidneys and colon, facilitating reduction of accumulated toxins. It is only available through health-care practitioners (see Resources).

*Milk Thistle (*Silybum marianum*)*

Milk thistle seed is a mild digestive bitter used in treating skin disorders and for cleansing the blood. Used since antiquity for digestive and liver complaints, it increases secretion and flow of bile. It gently promotes liver cleansing, but its primary actions go beyond. Milk thistle is known as one of the strongest liver herbs. It protects and regenerates the liver with its antioxidant properties by supporting RNA* synthesis, necessary for protein synthesis. It stimulates production of new liver cells and prevents formation of damaging leukotrienes.

Toxins that the liver neutralizes originate from within the body as well as from the outside world. During the cleansing process, the liver performs extra work—toxins are released from body tissues into the blood and lymph. Milk thistle protects liver

*RNA is a polymeric constituent of all living cells and many viruses. Its structure and base sequence of RNA are determinants of protein synthesis and the transmission of genetic information. Also called ribonucleic acid.

cells as they neutralize toxins by binding to them, and then dumps them into the colon for elimination. At the same time, it works hard to rebuild damaged liver tissue and also protects the kidneys.

The healing properties of milk thistle have been studied extensively for decades, primarily in Europe. Milk thistle has successfully treated patients with chronic hepatitis and cirrhosis; is active against hepatitis-B virus, and has shown to lower fat deposits in the liver of animals. Because of its blood-cleansing actions, milk thistle is also used for treating skin disorders such as psoriasis and eczema.

Note: The homeopathic formula described earlier as "RxDrainer" contains milk thistle and is much easier tolerated than the herbal form for hypersensitive individuals.

Blood Integrity—The Flow of Life

The Nectar of Rejuvenation

"Until man duplicates a blade of grass, Nature can laugh at his so-called scientific knowledge."
—Thomas A. Edison

Plant Life—Its Blood

According to a soil and plant scientist, Dr. G.H. Earp Thomas, green grasses like wheatgrass contain vital nutrients that serve as regenerative and protective factors within the body. His findings also concluded that its consumption is theoretically capable of sustaining human life for weeks, even months, at a time.

Wheatgrass juice has been referred to as "the blood of plant life" because it resembles the molecules of human red blood cells, transforming it into hemoglobin, which increases red blood cell count

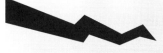

Flash-Back

Before I was introduced to organic wheatgrass juice concentrate, I didn't believe anything except fresh juice would provide the health benefits known for centuries. I grew flats of organic wheatgrass in my kitchen and sun room, only to react to the mold that formed in the soil from not maintaining perfect watering and climate controls.

To prove its effectiveness, I had a live cell microscopy blood test performed. The test allowed me to view my blood on a monitor along with the technician, as described in Chapter 6. I've had this type of blood test performed for over 10 years as a way to monitor overall health and make simple adjustments when needed.

I had the test performed before starting a daily protocol of fresh wheatgrass juice. I then juiced daily for 90 days and was retested. The results were amazing—the integrity (health) of my red blood cells was impressive!

To prove the effectiveness of organic, kosher, wheatgrass juice concentrate, I mixed one teaspoon in one ounce of spring water three times daily for the next 90 days and was again retested. The integrity of my blood cells was exactly the same as when consuming freshly squeezed juice. The red blood cells were "free-floating" with increased seed (oxygen) and the cellular membrane was healthier.

Because I had my blood tested prior to developing leaky gut, fibromyalgia, chronic fatigue and multiple allergic responses. I was a perfect candidate for testing the effectiveness that only live blood analysis confirms.

and the blood's capacity to deliver oxygen and other nutrients to the cell membrane. Chlorophyll, highly concentrated in wheatgrass juice, is similar in molecular structure to hemoglobin, the protein that carries oxygen to all the cells within the body.

Research scientists such as Dr. E. Bircher have come to respect the main constituent in wheatgrass juice, chlorophyll, as a body cleanser, rejuvenator, and neutralizer of toxins. With the emerging multitudes of invisible and chronic conditions like fibromyalgia, chronic fatigue, lupus, cancer, arthritis, digestive disorders and premature aging, to mention a few, our bodies need the health and rejuvenating benefits achieved from simply consuming one teaspoon of wheat grass juice concentrate in one-two ounces of water, two-three times a day.

Immune Enhancement—Supporting our Defenses

We know that our immune functions and the protection from infection and disease depend on the work of the white blood cells—providing the first-line of defense. Additionally, the body's ability to fight illness, including cancer, is determined by the strength of the immune system.

The late Dr. Ann Wigmore demonstrated the effectiveness of wheatgrass juice after decades of using it at her healing center in Boston. Wheatgrass juice, in contrast to modern drugs to correct one symptom or another without effectively strengthening the overall state of health, provides the necessary ingredients to strengthen the body's defenses for healing and regeneration. Wheatgrass juice acts as the body's healing weapon by providing concentrated ammunition to build defense arsenals against bacteria, viruses and, yes, even cancer.

Scientists confirm chlorophyll creates a health-enhancing intestinal environment by providing an eco-system that does not support the growth of health-depleting bacteria. By reducing and eliminating health-depleting bacteria, intestinal integrity remains strong—able to protect against disease-causing invaders.

"If only they knew, the use of grass is the most revolutionary concept introduced into the diet of society…In therapeutic amounts, wheatgrass internalizes a maximum of green chlorophyll and enzyme rich liquid food, to detoxify the body by increasing the elimination of hardened mucus, crystallized acids and solidified, decaying fecal matter. Its high enzyme content helps to dissolve tumors. It is the fastest surest way to eliminate internal waste and provide an optimum nutritional environment, so that the cosmic cell consciousness can rebuild your body." —Rev. Viktoras Kulvinskas, M.S., Survival into the 21st Century

Cell Regeneration—Charging our Battery

The substances found in roots of all young growing plants contain root auxins. In Dr. Ann Wigmore's

I was

Poisoned

by my body...

Since my recovery, I continue to consume two teaspoons of certified organic, kosher, wheatgrass juice concentrate daily, part of that in my special rejuvenation protein drink. Because of my extensive travel schedule, I use an additional "shot" on long flights and when I need that extra energy to fulfill my demanding schedule. I like using a one-ounce shot glass to get the actual sweet flavor of the juice.

I use and recommend Sheldon Farm wheatgrass juice because I'm aware that not all wheatgrass contains the same nutrients, depending on the way it's grown, nourished, harvested, juiced and freeze-dried. Sheldon Farm is greenhouse-grown and harvested year-around. It is grown in soil nourished with over 70 minerals and organic nutrients and freeze-dried at 50 degrees below zero to retain live-nutrient values. One teaspoon of wheatgrass juice concentrate contains the equivalent of 1 1/2 lbs. of raw organic vegetables (see Resources)!

writings, she cites research confirming experiments by botanists who "placed root auxins on the tip of a leaf, causing the root to grow on the edge of the leaf."

Further studies performed by the renowned Dr. Weston Price, founder of the Price-Pottenger Nutrition Foundation, isolated a substance from tips of young grasses which had a similar effect to that of root auxins, showing the ability of tender grasses to promote and regenerate damaged cells.

Wheatgrass contains such an abundance of natural, whole-food vitamins, minerals, trace elements, and enzymes that it is literally a source of energy producing fuel for the body. Because of its easy digestibility and rapid assimilation, it's a natural energy supplement whether alone or added to a protein-type supplement drink.

"15 lbs. of wheat grass is equal in overall nutritional value to 350 pounds of ordinary garden vegetables. We have not even scratched the surface of what grass can mean to man in the future." —Charles F. Schnabel, Agricultural Chemist, The Father of Wheat Grass

DNA Repair—Reproducing Healthy Cells

The general public is just now paying attention to the effects of reproduction within the DNA matrix. It has been scientifically verified that a compound (P4D1) found in young grasses has the ability to stimulate the production and natural repair of human reproductive sperm cells and DNA. A biologist at the University of California at San Diego, Dr. Yasuo Hotta tested reproductive cells. The following are his comments.

"Chlorophyll increases the functions of the heart, affects the vascular system, the intestines, the uterus, and the lungs. It raises the basic nitrogen exchange and is therefore a tonic which, considering its stimulating properties, cannot be compared with any other."

Enzymes—Life's Sustainability

Enzymes are essential for proper functioning of the body and are found in all living plant and animal matter. Their primary job is to maintain balanced body functions, digest food, and aid in the repair of tissue. Made up of proteins, thousands of identified enzymes play a critical role in virtually all body activities. *Life cannot be sustained without enzymes*, despite the presence of sufficient amounts of vitamins, minerals, water, and proteins. Scientists have been unable to manufacture enzymes synthetically. Each enzyme has a very specific biochemical function in the body, for which no other enzyme can be substituted.

According to Dr. Howard F. Loomis, Jr., "It is the enzymes that are responsible for the vast majority of all the biochemical reactions that bring our foods to maturity or ripeness." Enzymes are energy, and energy is defined in high school physics textbooks as the "capacity to do work." Enzymes are the electrical connectors driving metabolic functions. *Enzymes do not perform the work; rather they are the conductors.*

The shape of each specific enzyme is so specialized it initiates a reaction in only certain substances. Because enzymes are needed at various body sites, it's important efficiency is not reduced by overwork. A healthy body manufactures enzymes while maintaining its capacity to subsidize its supply obtained from food.

Unfortunately, enzymes are extremely sensitive to heat; even low temperatures will destroy them. To obtain enzymes from a food source, the food must be eaten raw (as in fresh vegetable or wheatgrass juice)—cooking or heating depletes *all* enzymes.

Digestive Enzymes—Their Functions

The primary work of digestive enzymes is to break down proteins, carbohydrates, and fats into smaller particles so the body can easily absorb nutrients through the stomach and small intestine. Digestion is primarily performed in the stomach and finished in the small intestine. The effect on intestinal microflora as a consequence of digestive efficiency includes stimulating the "good" bacteria in the gut, detoxifying and cleansing the colon, and improving digestive disorders that contribute to food and environmental allergies.

The body contains over 3,000 types of enzymes—many working in synchronicity with one another. Primary enzymes used for digestion include:

- Proteases—break down proteins (beef, chicken, poultry, fish, lamb, bison, etc.)
- Amylases—break down carbohydrates including starches (bread, pasta, potatoes, fruits, vegetables, sugars)
- Cellulase—breaks down cellulose (plant fiber), the indigestible part of fiber found in many fruits and vegetables
- Lipase—breaks down fats
- Papain (proteolytic enzyme)—breaks down proteins

- Bromelain (proteolytic enzyme)—breaks down proteins
- Maltase—breaks down malt sugar
- Lactose—breaks down milk sugar
- Invertase—breaks down sucrose (table sugar)

For highly sensitive individuals, I use and recommend four combinations in rotation that are very effective for LGS, MARS, EI and chronic disorders: Vital-Zymes® Forte, Zygest® and VegiZyme®, all professional formulas available through health-care practitioners (see Resources). My personal and professional experience has shown these complexes to be most helpful and least reactive.

After repair and recovery, I like to add, CapraZyme™, an enzyme blend that additionally contains herbs known to support a full spectrum of digestive functions.

Enzyme rotation is important because the body appears to become complacent if the same enzyme blend is used for prolonged periods. When hypersensitive, rotation as often as daily may be required. After recovery you may find, as I do, that rotating a bottle at a time is sufficient.

Note: The following is the protocol I find most effective in assuring a time-released-type action.

1. Consume a couple mouthfuls of food and then swallow one enzyme. Do not take on an empty stomach even though **none** of the formulas I use or recommend *contain hydrochloric acid* and all are vegetable enzymes.

2. At the end of the meal, swallow the second, allowing for a leisurely meal while assisting digestion until meal is completed.
3. Protein shakes and fresh juice are the same as consuming a meal. Follow above protocols.

Systemic Enzymes

Systemic enzymes are used for metabolic purposes in the bloodstream, unlike digestive enzymes used in the stomach and small intestine. Metabolic enzymes must be absorbed into the bloodstream in order to be effective. Enzymes made for systemic or metabolic functions are coated with an acid-resistant substance to prevent them from dissolving in stomach acid. The next section provides an in-depth look at systemic metabolic enzymes and their uses.

Note: Systemic enzymes should be taken on an empty stomach, *at least 45 minutes before or after eating.*

"I Hurt All Over"—The Drug Alternative for Pain and Inflammation

When our bodies are unable to deal with toxic overload, the reaction is pain and inflammation. Many illnesses, and nearly all injuries, result in inflammatory responses to various degrees, supporting the methodology that there exists a common denominator in LGS, inflammatory disorders, and immune system dysfunction. This common denominator is evident in related conditions such as

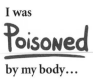
fibromyalgia, chronic fatigue, lupus, arthritis, and myofascial pain syndrome. It is estimated that 26,000,000 people, in the U.S. alone, have fibromyalgia, myofascial pain syndrome, or both. That figure is alarming to me, and it should be to you.

When the immune system malfunctions and becomes hyperactive, it over-reacts and produces antibodies that attack even harmless substances in the blood. This action causes formation of irritating circulating immune complexes (CICs); so misshapen and foreign to the body, they themselves are attacked by the immune system. Otherwise healthy tissues in the same neighborhood may also be affected causing further exacerbation of the immune response; the immune system attacks the body's own cells and tissues, resulting in chronic pain and inflammation.

Most conventional treatments address symptoms of inflammation with anti-inflammatory medications, not addressing the underlying systemic condition. These medications initially reduce pain and inflammation but, in the process, cause dangerous side-effects and do nothing to start the healing process. I know—**I've Done That Already** (IDTA)!

Systemic oral enzymes stimulate healthy production of messenger immune cells (cytokines). These reduce inflammation and speed up immunity by producing a cleansing effect and helping to break up CICs at the center of the body's immune/inflammation response.

The effects of systemic oral enzyme therapy on the immune system and treatment of auto-immune diseases, especially rheumatoid factors, are profound and may involve intense therapy for weeks or months. Remember, we're dealing with causes of the disorder, not *suppressing* or *masking* the symptoms. If you're in acute pain, your physician can assist you in incorporating prescription drugs (for immediate relief) with enzyme therapy (for long-term healing).

Systemic Enzymes—Their Benefits
- degrades protein molecules penetrating from blood capillaries into tissues—causing edema and exacerbation of inflammatory processes
- increases flexibility of red blood cells—improving their ability to pass through capillaries
- inhibits aggregation of platelets
- degrades cell fragments—mediators of inflammation and infection
- increases fibrinolytic activities in the blood—helping to prevent abnormal clotting
- activates white blood cells (macrophages), natural killer cells—better equipping immune system to deal with inflammation by cleansing itself of cellular debris and quickly neutralizing errant cancer cells
- supports cleansing of tissues and promotes better circulation
- stimulates formation of new, healthy tissue

Systemic enzyme therapy markedly reduces the body's inflammation level, enabling the person to once again resume normal activity and restore quality of life, *Naturally*.

I reviewed hundreds of pages on systemic oral enzymes and used several dozen brands. The one product that is responsible for eliminating my chronic muscle pain and inflammation and facilitating rejuvenation is Wobenzym N®, manufactured in Germany by the Mucos Pharma GmbH & Co. Recent research confirms it is now recognized as the most effective systemic enzyme blend in the world. Wobenzym N is endorsed by leading European scientists and is backed by over 30 years of scientific research and clinical studies confirming its benefits.

Why hasn't your health-care provider recommended systemic oral enzymes instead of drugs with their side-effects?

Sadly, conventional health-care providers may not know about the benefits of systemic oral enzymes. European studies are not totally validated as a basis for clinical opinion in the U.S. Our U.S. medical education system tends to not teach nutrition—teaching only the bare basics about the use of vitamin and mineral therapies. Most American medical journals have, until recently, avoided articles on nutrition, feeling they should be published elsewhere or not at

all. It appears that a great majority of doctors seem
uncomfortable recommending a food or natural
substance rather than drugs. It is notable the position is beginning to change.

Our economy is now global, as are resources for
products. Multi-national clinical trials are becoming more abundant and the information on medicine and therapies is now as close as your computer.
The European and Asian research is as good, if not
better, than the research done in America. It is my
opinion that systemic oral enzymes offer the first
mainstream long-term treatment option for

Flash-Forward

FACILITATING REJUVENATION— MANAGING PAIN AND INFLAMMATION

The goal must be not only to manage pain and inflammation, but also to provide natural support for bones, ligaments,
tendons, and connective tissues—not an easy task for a non-
pharmaceutical product. The product I use and recommend
for these purposes is a complete, comprehensive bone and
joint support formula, containing Type II chicken collagen
(free-ranged—free of growth hormones, antibiotics, pesticides and insecticides). It additionally contains cartilage and
bone-building nutrients to provide the body what it needs to
increase bone density while rebuilding healthy cartilage and
connective tissue. Collagen also stimulates production of the
cells responsible for maintaining joint-cushioning cartilage—
important in both repair and maintenance as we age.
CapraFlex™ is the only blend I use and recommend that
includes four synergistically balanced blends all in one caplet:
Osteo-enhancing, Joint and Cartilage Matrix, ArthriFlex, and
Anti-inflammatory blends (see Resources).

inflammatory disorders, with proven healing and safety—particularly true when compared to corticosteroids and non-steroidal anti-inflammatory drugs (NSAIDs) with their side-effects, of which I am a prime example.

I began by taking 10 Wobenzym N tablets three times a day on an empty stomach. The tablets are about the size of a commonly recognized round, candy-coated chocolate, without the coloring agent. The results were the same as when I took the NSAIDs. I now take a maintenance dose of five tablets two times a day. My clients report similar results and keep saying, "Why didn't someone tell me about systemic enzymes before now?" You be the judge (see Resources).

Parasites—Eliminating Your Unwanted House Guests

You may be shocked to know what medical experts say about parasites:

"85% of adult North Americans are infected with parasites."—Dr. Hazel Parcels

"In terms of numbers, more parasitic infections are acquired in the U.S. than in Africa." –Dr. Frank Nova, Chief of the Laboratory for Parasitic Diseases of the U.S. National Institute of Health

"I believe the single most undiagnosed health challenge in the history of the human race is parasites."—Dr. Ross Anderson

It is my experience that most people with gastrointestinal disorders, inflammatory diseases (such as arthritis and fibromyalgia), skin disorders, and allergies have parasites—especially evident in cases of LGS and irritable bowel syndrome. Most people *falsely* believe they don't have to concern themselves with the possibility of parasites if they haven't visited another country or traveled far from home. Nothing is further from the truth.

According to a report published by *The Environmental Working Group* in Washington, D.C., most municipal water systems in the U.S. are homes to protozoa (a single-cell organism that can only divide within a host organism) like *Giardia* and *Cryptosporidium*. The group also reported that one in five Americans drinks water that violates federal health standards. Every year, nearly a million North Americans become sick from waterborne diseases; one percent dies.

Types of worms living in the gastrointestinal tract include, but are not limited to, tapeworm, threadworm, roundworm, pinworm, and hookworm.

Treatment for removal of parasitic infection is not a do-it-yourself project. There are many forms of natural therapies that do not produce the side-effects of drug therapies and are often more effective. One important fact to keep in mind, however, is that repeated therapies are sometimes required to achieve complete success. If you have a prolonged digestive disorder, you should consider having a comprehensive parasitology screening (described in Chapter 6), before proceeding with a parasite cleanse under the direction of a health-care professional.

Natural remedies work effectively, as evidenced by re-testing; however, you must remain on the therapy program for an initial 8-12 weeks and repeat as directed. After initial detoxification, I recommend a maintenance parasite cleanse for two weeks twice a year.

Intestinal Housecleaning

Specifically in LGS, parasites have a perfect gastrointestinal environment in which to thrive: warm, dark, damp, and toxic. The first step is to cleanse the gastrointestinal tract with a quality colon fiber cleanse complex. It is necessary to brush the lining of the intestinal wall, ridding the body of parasites that are well established and attached. If this step is not taken, parasite remedies will not be effective because they cannot reach the worms until the encrusted waste matter and mucus protecting the worms are loosened or removed. This encrustation becomes a cozy protective housing for the parasites and must be removed to get to the core of the infestation.

Once you begin a colon fiber cleanse you will most likely pass thick strings of mucus, worms, and putrefied fecal matter. By removing these substances you are destroying the habitat protecting these unwanted guests.

Parasitic Therapies—Natural Solutions

My experiences with clients prove that most hypersensitive individuals cannot tolerate complexes that contain standard herbal formulas until initial reduction of toxic load is accomplished. However, best tolerated and effective protocols include a homeopathic parasite cleanse, combined with a specific enzyme blend, for an initial 12-week cleanse as outlined:

- **Weeks 1 & 2**—one dropper-full (as much as the dropper will hold) of a homeopathic "Parasite" liquid complex in a small amount of water two times daily on an empty stomach*
- **Week 3**—take the same homeopathic complex as weeks 1 & 2 plus two capsules of Zymex® II, a professional enzyme blend of five enzymes, defatted almond nut, and fig*
- **Weeks 4 & 5**—repeat weeks 1 & 2 above*
- **Weeks 6 & 7**—take only Zymex II, two capsules twice a day*
- **Weeks 8 & 9**—take only two droppers-full of homeopathic twice a day in water*
- **Weeks 10 & 11**—take two droppers-full twice a day of homeopathic along with two Zymex II capsules twice a day*
- **Week 12**—take only two Zymex II twice a day*

*Definition of an empty stomach: *45 minutes before or after eating food. Water and noncaffeinated teas do not constitute food.*

Note: If you are extremely reactive, you may have to start with 1-3 drops of the homeopathic in water and slowly increase. Do not count the start of your protocol until you're able to follow the above recommendations (see resource guide for both professional products).

Parasitic Therapies—Conventional Approach

Drug therapies can be effective; however, one must weigh the benefits against the adverse effects from the toxicity of such drugs. In the book, *Guess What Came to Dinner*, Ann Louise Gittleman, Ph.D., provides a comprehensive list of anti-parasitic drugs and their side-effects. The list includes physician references from *The Medical Letter on Drugs and Therapeutics*. Anyone desiring to expand his or her knowledge of parasitic infections would benefit from reading this detailed and well-referenced book.

Today, the conventional medical single-drug-course cure rate is less than 5%, and approximately half of the patients treated with drugs such as Flagyl® (metronidazole) complain of side-effects and refuse to take it again. Because of the low percentage of successful eradication with drugs, some physicians are now choosing to refer patients to natural health professionals for individualized natural detoxification protocols. These therapies are proven safer, gentler, and generally more effective.

As previously mentioned, there are two effective ways to flush out old fecal matter, *Candida,* and parasites: professional colon hydro-therapy and enemas—assisted by the consumption of colon fiber cleanses. It is important to remember that as parasites are loosened, they must be fully eliminated so they don't add to the toxic load. Colon hydro-therapy cleanses the entire length of the colon, all the way to the ileocecal valve, located at the juncture of the small and large intestines. Enemas only reach the lower $12^1/2$ inches of the $5^1/2$-foot-long colon. The type of therapy will depend on the recommendation from a health-care practitioner, financial considerations, and availability of qualified colon hydro-therapists in your area (see Resources).

During any cleansing process, it's inevitable some of the probiotics (health-enhancing microorganisms) are also eliminated. Be sure to check with your health-care professional as to quantity and type of probiotics best suited for your needs.

Diet and Parasites

According to most dietary experts, a diet high in simple carbohydrates like sugar, white flour, and processed foods, provides the perfect environment for feeding parasites and yeast.

We know that fiber-deficient foods precipitate a breeding ground for parasites, requiring a longer transit time to pass through the alimentary system. Slow transit time allows more food to decay and putrefy—producing stagnation in the colon that sets up the perfect living conditions for parasites and *Candida* to thrive.

The challenge for victims of LGS is that their diet must contain the foods they tolerate without allergic responses. Therefore, I will refrain from giving specific dietary recommendations regarding a parasitic cleansing diet, because it must be designed specifically for each individual by a qualified natural health professional.

Natural Relief from Nausea

Some patients experience slight nausea during the die-off of parasites. This symptom is generally experienced because of the toxic by-products released by the parasites into the body. There are several effective natural substances that provide relief.

1. Homeopathic dilution of ipecac syrup causes no adverse side-effects and is successful in dealing with nausea. Concentrated ipecac syrup has been used for years to induce vomiting. The homeopathic dilution has the reverse effect. Be sure to check with a health-care practitioner for proper dosage and potency.

2. Aloe vera juice distillate is another natural substance that provides immediate relief from nausea (refer to specifics for selecting aloe juice, previously discussed).

3. Ginger extract is excellent for nausea. Place several drops in a glass of warm water and sip slowly. Fresh ginger tea is also effective, but does not bring relief as fast as extract dilution. It is sold in most health food stores and select pharmacies.

Note: the more nausea you experience, the more parasitic infection you have.

Depositing Reserves in Your pH Immune Account

Your saliva pH is a measurement of the alkaline/acid condition of your body. Maintaining an optimal pH level is essential for activating the digestive juices. The neutral pH is between 7.0 and 7.2. Keeping the body slightly alkaline discourages fungus, mold, *Candida*, and parasites—all thriving in an acidic environment. According to the late Dr. Bernard Jensen, the optimum pH for human tissue and blood plasma ranges from 7.35 to 7.45. As an example, distilled water has a pH of 7.0. Water pH can vary greatly depending on the source. The water in a valley in Washington State has a pH of 8.5 because of abundant basalt base rock.

If the body is too acid or too alkaline, illness and disease will likely escalate. You can perform a pH test easily and economically at home by purchasing test strips available through a pharmacist. With LGS, it is best to test urine (not saliva) first thing in the morning with the first voiding. Your pH should maintain somewhere between 6.8 and 7.2.

A great deal of misconception exists about what is acid and what is alkaline. The acid-alkaline action is not necessarily related to how foods taste; citrus fruits taste acidic and are alkaline-forming.

An alkaline ecosystem (intestinal flora) will create an unfriendly environment for uninvited organisms. Your diet should consist of 70%-80% alkaline-forming foods. It is also helpful to eat 50% of your daily food raw—allowing for full benefits of enzymes, otherwise destroyed by cooking or heating.

At the onset of LGS, raw food other than in juices is not generally tolerated. Go slowly and pay attention to your response. As your gut heals you'll be able to tolerate more and more raw foods.

The following is a basic guide to the acid- and alkaline-producing food groups:

- **Vegetables**—All vegetables are alkaline-forming, including high-carbohydrate foods like potatoes, squash, and parsnips.
- **Grain**—Most grains are acid-forming, except millet and buckwheat. Seeds and grains become more alkaline-forming if sprouted.
- **Vegetable and fruit juices**—Most vegetable and fruit juices are highly alkaline-forming. Berry juices such as huckleberry, raspberry, blackberry, elderberry, boysenberry, and currents are all alkaline-forming. However, strawberries and cranberries are acid-forming.

- **Sugars**—All sugars are acid-forming with the exception of honey, which is alkaline-forming.
- **Meats, fish and dairy products** are all acid-forming with the exception of sheep and goat products, which generally have an alkaline reaction.

Emotional Support

My intent is to share first-hand information to assist you, and those who care about you, to regain a quality of life in a society that lives to eat, not eats to live. Is it easy? No. Is it possible? *Yes.*

Surviving in a Society that Revolves Around Eating

One of the most challenging aspects of living with multiple allergic responses is the potential social isolation as a result of traditions revolving around eating. The history of gathering for a meal goes back two million years when Protohominid hunters and foragers shared food with their fellow hunters and their families. When we eat together, we bring along our culture, customs, and expectations—providing us a way of communicating and sharing. Eating becomes not just a "food event," but also an event with complex challenges for the person with leaky gut syndrome (LGS) and/or multiple allergic response syndrome (MARS). However, the challenges lie in adjusting our attitudes and the attitudes of those with whom we socialize.

Having to modify our eating surely does not have to keep people apart. On the contrary, it can be an opportunity to individualize and create new food events. It's a time to reflect and acknowledge our need to communicate—the true essence of gathering in the first place. It's a time for us to ask our social family for support in treating us as "normal," not as a person with a contagious disease. People with eating disorders are not contagious; they simply have specific requirements for the food they can safely consume. We are physically challenged, not emotionally impaired, even though at times you wonder if "your emotional goat cheese slipped off its rice cracker!"

Allergies and allergic responses can be a divisive and isolating force in our society if we allow them to be. Be specific in asking for what you need from social situations. Express a desire to be included in gatherings and bring your own food. Ask people close to you to refrain from attempts to convince you to "just have a little, it can't hurt." Explain that you understand they may feel awkward or even guilty consuming foods you can't. Assure them it's their companionship that's important to you, not what you consume. Add some humor; tell them you're participating in a new food event called "name that food."

Be prepared to encounter individuals who were never challenged with food allergies and who will say (or think) you're downright neurotic, especially when they observe you eating foods they don't recognize

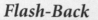

Flash-Back

The first Thanksgiving holiday after the onset of my illness was the most challenging. I invited 12 guests for my traditional formal, sit-down dinner. My youngest son was coming home to spend the holiday for the first time in years. I was determined to fix a full dinner, even though I was unable to eat anything on the menu. I was still on a very limited diet, and I didn't want to risk an allergic response from a newly introduced food. It was important to me to proceed with plans, regardless of my health challenges. It's not my style, or consciousness, to focus on my limitations, but it was quite challenging as a gourmet cook to prepare the entire meal and not be able to taste as I cooked.

One of my guests, an art teacher, inquired beforehand as to what I could eat. "Organic carrots, rice, and apples," I responded.

When time came to sit down to a full complement of food, she presented me with a work of art. She and her daughter had shredded organic carrots and sculptured an absolutely beautiful turkey. It filled the dinner plate, complete with eyes and anatomical details. I was overwhelmed! The focus of the dinner became the masterpiece of my carrot turkey, not my limitations. Thanks to the thoughtfulness and sensitivity of special friends, I too enjoyed my holiday turkey made from carrots, an example of the true meaning of Thanksgiving—sharing and giving thanks, especially thanks for the kindness extended by caring friends.

and usually can't pronounce. To those individuals, simply say, "I'm happy you have never experienced severe allergies and I hope you never do." It is curious that eventually people start asking about the nonconventional foods you're consuming. This provides a perfect opportunity to embark in new conversations, expanding their horizons, vocabulary, and hopefully, their emotional sensitivity to those with special needs. These occasions provide you an opportunity to bring something new to the dining table—knowledge of what you eat, and why you eat it.

Asking for What You Need— Help Others Help You

For some of us, asking for help is extremely difficult. Fortunately, I have a personal support system like none I've ever witnessed or encountered—not everyone is as blessed. The following components were, for me, the most important in structuring my support team: acknowledgement, validation, privacy, and education.

Acknowledge the Fear

Fear as described by *Webster's* is "an unpleasant often strong emotion caused by anticipation or awareness of danger...Fear is the most general term and implies anxiety and usually loss of courage (fear of the unknown)."

At the onset of any illness, fear was the first human response. LGS, MARS/EI, and fibromyalgia are not acknowledged or understood by most conventional professionals, much less in your personal support team. Be patient. Acknowledge your fear; it's the first step in coping with it. Express your concerns to your support team; it's the only way they can assist in diminishing some of your fears. It's amazing how some fears are monumental to us, yet to the support team, they seem so basic, especially when your supporters know what they're dealing with.

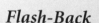

Flash-Back

My fears were, "Will I suffocate by not being able to swallow"? "What if I'm driving and I have a reaction?" "Where will I find the foods I can tolerate?" "I don't have enough energy to go shopping, much less locate specialty items." "Why don't my adult children understand this is life-threatening?"

My primary concern was finding a source of organic foods in the middle of winter in northern Idaho. I didn't have the energy to travel great distances in search of specialty sources. When I mentioned my dilemma to a client who had become a friend, she immediately replied, "I go into the city (125 miles away) every two weeks. I'd be happy to shop for whatever you need," and…the personal shopper was created. Before long, I had friends and clients using her services as well. This single mother of three found a need, filled it, and supplemented her income. She transformed regular trips to a large city into a service for others who are challenged by poor health, lack of time, and/or adequate transportation.

Privacy

According to Webster's, privacy is "the quality or state of being apart from company or observation."

Sometimes emotional support simply means giving you more space. This is especially evident when your body is experiencing so many physical changes and requires special considerations on a daily basis. It's not like you drink juice in the morning, take your supplements and you're okay for the rest of the day. You are forced to embark on a 24-hour-a-day challenge, a complete life-style change.

Explain to the people around you that sometimes you just need to have personal quiet time to reflect, heal, and take stock of your situation. It is not helpful for someone like a well-meaning neighbor, friend, or relative to chat, visit, or ask for daily reports on your condition—energy we just don't have to give. I assess situations by asking, "Is this experience going to be a taker or giver of energy?" If the situation is too energy-consuming then I gracefully bow out or become unavailable. There may be situations when you need to express that the best

Flash-Back

The first few months were so challenging I had to detach from well-meaning friends and neighbors. I was in colon hydro-therapy 2-3 times a week, maintained a limited consulting practice, delved into medical research and writing, had therapeutic massage and lymphatic stimulation weekly, juiced daily, and experimented with every food and food preparation method I could get my hands on. Living became overwhelming, a full-time job, while I faced the challenges with less energy than I'd ever experienced.

help comes in the form of simply giving you space.

People outside your household who can't, or don't choose to, contribute by assisting in daily necessary tasks, (shopping for organic foods, preparing food for juicing, cooking, etc.) should be emotionally supportive by respecting your need for space. If you agree to anything less, you'll pay the huge price of adding toxic emotions of disappointment, anxiety, and resentment to your already toxic body.

Education and Validation

Educating is to "provide with information" (*Webster's*). Ask those who care about you to read all they can regarding digestive disorders, food allergies, *Candida*, parasites, drug side-effects, multiple allergic responses, environmental illness, and particularly, to read this book by a professional "who's been there." Explain the choices you've made in taking control of your health-care. Give them permission to disagree with your decisions, all the while communicating your request for them to respect your decisions. If they choose to continue pressing their point of view, don't feed their negativity. If asked, be willing to provide background material and suggested reading so they may better understand your challenges and needs. Usually, the people quickest to express an opinion are the ones least informed. *To the uninformed, anything less than drug therapy must be "quackery."* It soon becomes evident these people know nothing of alternative natural healing modalities used and written about for centuries. They are accustomed to quick fixes. Wholistic medicine is not quick. It is effective and the investment pays higher dividends than symptom-care and drug-management. Make it clear you are not asking permission, you are expressing a decision. If they choose not to be supportive, respect their position, fade out of their life, and find a new support team. It's better to be alone than with someone who is not supportive or is outright critical.

Many individuals, clients and non-clients, contacted me when they heard I was writing about leaky gut syndrome, fibromyalgia, and the resulting multiple chemical sensitivities and allergic responses. I was consistently asked to write about guidance in dealing with people who are not informed about natural health and have no idea about the seriousness of these conditions. Their suggestions, blended with my experiences, helped to formulate this chapter. I am honored they chose to share their stories of personal challenge, and thankful to the thousands who have allowed me into their lives to assist them on their journey to wellness, *Naturally*.

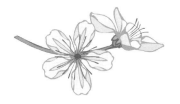

Living with the Effects of Leaky Gut Syndrome (LGS) and Multiple Allergic Response Syndrome (MARS)

Reaction-Emergency Preparedness

EACH PERSON has individual responses and needs. Do not attempt to control allergic reactions without the assistance and ongoing support of your physician and natural health-care practitioner.

An allergic response can begin suddenly, peaking within minutes, or develop gradually over hours or days. Death can occur because patients, or those around them, do not recognize or validate the severity of the allergic response. Prolonged stressful respiratory restriction is challenging for the functioning of the entire body. You must begin to manage the attack at the *earliest sign* of reaction.

- Have a plan worked out with your physician, health-care practitioner, and those close to you on how to handle an emergency.

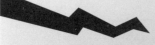

- Be sure to update your medical consent or durable power of attorney for healthcare. Keep a copy with you at all times and make a note of its location on any identification you carry with you.
- Give copies of your medical consent to everyone authorized to make decisions on your behalf.
- Alert family members, co-workers, close friends, and neighbors about your condition.
- Be specific regarding your needs, what action to take, and who to contact if an allergic response occurs.
- If someone does not take your condition seriously, don't try to convince them, ask someone else.
- Wear a medical alert bracelet or necklace; it may save your life.

How I "Get Out" of Allergic Responses

I use the following steps to "get out" of allergic responses to food or environmental causes, *Naturally*:

Flash-Back

Before my recovery, my kit contained emergency injectable epinephrine (Adrenaline) and an inhaler, prescribed by my medical doctor. I never used the epinephrine—the homeopathic remedy was successful in controlling my reactions. I did use the inhaler at the onset of my leaky gut, until an effective natural remedy could be identified and the overall toxic load in my body was reduced. When in a reactive state, I immediately notified someone close to me in the event I couldn't speak for myself—which you should always do if experiencing any type of allergic response or reaction.

1. I remove myself from the suspected food or pollutant immediately.

   If ingested—I discontinue eating the food or substance.

   If environmental—I get out immediately into clean,
fresh air and proceed to step 2 and 3.

2. If possible, at first sign of an allergic response, I
dissolve one teaspoon of a high potency Vitamin C
powder in warm water and swallow (room temperature water is fine if that's all that's handy). The
one I use is a professional brand called Ultra
Potent C Powder®. One teaspoon contains 4,350
mg. I pre-measure a teaspoon and carry it, well
labeled, in a small glass vial (see Resources).

3. I use a homeopathic remedy specifically for allergic responses (see Resources). I administer six
drops directly under the tongue and repeat every
5-8 minutes, as needed. The immediate emergency

Living with
the Effects of
Leaky Gut
Syndrome (LGS)
and Multiple
Allergic Response
Syndrome
(MARS)

Flash-Forward

Ten years later, my emergency response kit
contains:

✓ a lightweight mask called "I can breathe™" with a disposable charcoal filter in the event I encounter a situation that
is not environmentally safe (see Resources for mask)

✓ 1 tsp. Ultra Potent C powder or caplets

✓ homeopathic for allergic reactions

✓ Benedryl®—in the event I need relief for several hours
before assistance or supplies are available

reaction subsides after first dose, the total allergic response usually after 3-4 doses.

Note: You should always *carry these two items to assist with allergic responses. Some clients are forced to additionally carry an inhaler, oxygen, and injectable epinephrine prescribed by their physician, as I did at the onset of my illness.*

4. If the reaction is from an environmental source, I shower and wash my hair at the first opportunity. This is critical to minimize absorption of the offending substance and reduce toxic overload.

5. After an acute reaction, it's important to cleanse the gastrointestinal tract; I perform colon hydro-therapy as soon as possible. I'm fortunate to now have access to a professional colon-hydrotherapy machine and a therapist at my request. There were times when I had to call the therapist and exclaim, "I'm having an acute reaction, I'm on my way." As soon as colon therapy was administered, my reactions disappeared. If I'm not able to have colon hydro-therapy, I administer enemas. Enemas provide some reaction relief, but cannot compare to the immediate relief of colon hydro-therapy.

6. After an acute reaction I maintain a liquid diet for 1-2 days. The diet consists of fresh juices, my special rejuvenation protein drink, and herbal teas. This regimen allows the body systems to use the energy for detoxifying and repair by giving the digestive system a rest.

261

Living with
the Effects of
Leaky Gut
Syndrome (LGS)
and Multiple
Allergic Response
Syndrome
(MARS)

7. I take additional Vitamin C to bowel tolerance (the dose tolerated before developing diarrhea). It assists in boosting the immune system by producing lymphocytes. Vitamin C prevents free-radical damage and is used by the thymus gland (involved in immunity) to increase the mobility of phagocyte cells, which "eat" bacteria, viral cells, and other harmful foreign substances. Normally I take 4000mg as a total daily dose. I take higher levels of vitamin C for 3-4 days after an acute reaction. For the LGS patient, it's important to find individual tolerance levels and to always take vitamin C with food. Taking it on an empty stomach may cause stomach or G.I. discomfort (see Resources for Ultra Potent C powder or caplets).

8. I increase my consumption of a complete vitamin B complex with folic acid. I take a daily total of 200mg of B complex (which includes 400mcg of folic acid per 100mg). I continue this for seven days, and then return to my maintenance dose of one 100mg tablet daily, with meals. Vitamin B plays an important role in the health of the gastrointestinal tract and nervous system, is needed for healthy blood, and produces red blood cells and antibodies. Folic acid assists the immune system by increasing the ability to recognize invading microbes and strengthening white blood cells.

9. I use a unique air sterilizer called Life Pro™ with a six-stage filtration system in my home, office, and

car. Life Pro is proven to kill most airborne pathogens and allergy-causing contaminants. Units similar to these have been used successfully by the military to protect soldiers against multiple airborne pathogens of unknown origin (see Resources). The one for my car is also adaptable to carry while traveling for use in hotel rooms, etc. When I fly, I place the travel unit in its carrying case in my checked luggage.

10. I stay in my "safe" areas (home and office) for a few days, until all lingering effects of the allergic

Flash-Forward

I no longer react with anaphylactic reactions; however, I never let my guard down . I no longer use a mask while flying, but carry one just in case. I haven't used the oxygen tank in over eight years, but still keep it updated as added security.

Recently, I was on a flight whose departure was delayed for over an hour while the aircraft was in line for takeoff on the tarmac; the jet fuel was being "sucked" into the cabin. I started to feel my face get hot and welt. I immediately grabbed my vitamin C powder, dissolved it in water, and took it. I then put six drops of my homeopathic remedy for allergic reactions under my tongue and put on my mask.

Several people around me were also feeling ill from the fumes and many commented they wish they were as well prepared. If they only knew what I'd been through to get to this point of preparedness! I have experienced only two serious allergic responses within the last five years, but I don't put myself in toxic environments if I know in advance. The four items I carry with me take up less room than a comb and handkerchief. In this toxic world of unknowns, it's prudent to always be prepared!

response have disappeared. This is imperative because the body needs time to detoxify and repair.

11. Most of all, I do whatever I can to reduce stress and stressful situations. Stress, combined with a reaction, compromises the already overworked immune system by adding to your total accumulated exposure (TAE).

12. I lower my expectations and allow my body time to recuperate. At first, it was difficult to grant myself permission to slow down. My mind was operating at the usual fast pace, but my body couldn't keep up. This situation encouraged me to create the phrase, "My mind is writing checks my body can't cash"…humor is great medicine.

Note: I also have a portable oxygen tank in my office and home. This is critical if an environmental exposure occurs and emergency measures are needed—also valuable for clearing acute "brain-fog." Check with your health-care provider; he/she will guide you in acquiring a tank, precautions, and proper dosage.

263

Living with
the Effects of
Leaky Gut
Syndrome (LGS)
and Multiple
Allergic Response
Syndrome
(MARS)

My Battered Ration Crate

Travel, for most of us, is inevitable. Travel has a significant meaning in each person's life-style. For the purposes of this book, I'll deal with everyday travel as required to and from our place of employment and everyday necessities. Traveling abroad or for long distances requires careful advance planning and special accommodations.

During my illness, my business partner creatively assembled a plastic crate with a tight fitting cover for my on-the-go food. Some of the items I found invaluable include:

- Brown rice cakes
- Brown rice crackers
- Almonds or nuts (as tolerated)
- Goat-milk protein powder
- Spoon, fork, small spreading knife, small sharp knife
- Glass canning jar and lid (to use as shaker for protein drink)
- Small bowl and plate (wood or ceramic)
- Small stainless box for digestive enzymes (see my website for hinged-stainless boxes)
- Small containers of organic applesauce or any tolerated organic baby food

Flash-Back

I've experienced panic at being away from my food sources when I can't get home soon enough to keep my body from experiencing a negative reaction. I remember having to make a trip to a major city some 125 miles away. I thought I packed enough food for the day. All the appointments took much longer than anticipated, and by early evening I was out of food. The health-food stores were closed and restaurants weren't an option. I finally resorted to buying some rice milk and rice cakes from an all-night grocery store. No, it wasn't a meal, but it got me through the emergency. That incident was what encouraged my business partner to assemble the "on-the-go" crate for me—never again placing myself in a situation without my basic needs.

- Small single-serving containers of rice, almond, or hazelnut milk (these do not require refrigeration until opened)
- Individual servings of organic juices (as tolerated)
- Plenty of napkins
- Small bags to use for garbage
- Bottles of pure drinking water
- A washcloth in a plastic bag

Being a native Californian, we call kits like these "earthquake survival kits." In Idaho they're called "snow survival kits." A kit like this would be a great start for general "emergency preparedness"—same purpose, taking care of your needs when other resources are not readily available. Even if you don't live in a rural area as I do, it's not always convenient to locate a store with an organic food department at the time you need it. For those of us with food allergies and allergic responses, the challenge is not only finding the foods we can tolerate; they must be organic—a profound difference. Being prepared is essential, it puts us *back in control*, and that's important at a time when everything in our health and environment is so out of control.

My Battered Ice Chest

It's a good thing I drive a sport utility vehicle because I need room for my supplies. An ice chest is another necessity when traveling away from home. Since you'll probably be cooking extra quantities of food for your trip, whether a few hours or several days, it's important to properly store it. Avoid experiencing food-borne illnesses from improper refrigeration and the resulting bacteria.

I have a client who had dinner at a restaurant on a hot August day, and took home the leftovers (without an ice chest). The trip home was 30 minutes and the car was air-conditioned.

Upon arriving home, she immediately refrigerated the leftover food. The following evening she decided to eat the leftovers. Later that night the effects of food poisoning hit: acute stomach pain, vomiting, and diarrhea, requiring a trip to the emergency room and I.V. therapy. That dinner cost her over $1,200 and created a potentially life-threatening situation. Isn't an ice chest and some ice worth the small investment? Someone with a weakened digestive and immune system acquiring food poisoning could truly be indulging in their *last supper*. Whatever foods you are currently tolerating, cook extra quantities and carry some with you and keep them cold.

Business and Overnight Trips

I have many clients who, like me, travel extensively for business. They resort to carrying a soft-sided insulated chest as part of their allowed carry-on luggage. The prepared foods are previously frozen and act as the cooling agent. Planning ahead allows them to *fit* into a normal life-style.

When obtaining lodging, be sure to ask if they have facilities to warm and refrigerate food. If the facility has a restaurant, ask to speak with the food service manager or chef. Explain your special dietary needs—most facilities will accommodate your requests. Also inquire if they would cook for you if you provide the food. It's amazing what you get if you just ask for it! Don't be embarrassed; millions of people have special dietary and environmental needs, and establishments are more and more willing to cooperate. Carrying or purchasing your own food allows you to travel with confidence, assured of the ingredients.

The following suggestions for traveling are my personal preferences and those submitted by clients:

- *Frozen organic vegetables*—peas, green beans, spinach, chard, corn, bean sprouts, celery, chopped onions, and garlic. I shop and freeze small bags of onions and minced or juiced frozen garlic, to add to stir fries and omelets. Be sure to freeze in small quantities for a single meal.
- *Frozen cooked grains*—brown rice, brown basmati rice, quinoa, teff. Don't overcook for freezing—leave it a little al dente. When reheated it can be stir fried or steamed. Place just enough grain in a bag for a single serving.
- *Frozen spinach or veggie patties*—I make delectable chard patties (sautéed onions, chard, garlic, rice bread crumbs, egg, one packet of SweetLife, chopped

nuts, herbs) and pan-fry in coconut oil. They are a great hot main course and just as tasty cold. I've served them to guests who can't believe they're eating a meatless patty.

Get creative. Turn your necessity into a new gourmet experience. You may be pleasantly surprised by the curiosity expressed and the interesting conversations that result, *Naturally*.

Flash-Forward

I no longer carry my food on trips, except for long flights when I still make my veggie patties because they're delicious cold and easily packed into my carry-on luggage. I eat in restaurants and carefully explain my needs to the food server or chef. I do not eat in fast-food establishments because I know their food is purchased in bulk and contains ingredients to enhance flavors and extend shelf-life.

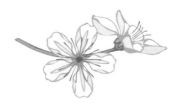

Afterword

MODERN CONVENTIONAL MEDICINE performs miracles and saves lives, especially in the case of injury or trauma. I'm a prime example; clot-dissolving drugs saved my life after a traumatic injury. Doctors perform daily miracles by repairing physical damage and removing (and often replacing) diseased organs and limbs. However, conventional medicine has little to offer an individual with digestive disorders, multiple allergic response syndrome (MARS), environmental illnesses (EI), and chronic disorders. Physicians are trained to "turn off" a reaction with drugs for symptom-care and, in the process, perpetuate a self-destructive cycle masking the root causes.

A new breed of health-care practitioners and physicians employ methods advocated by Hippocrates. They emphasize diet, nutrients, non-toxic treatments, environmental modifications, and therapies that encourage the healing process—reserving drugs and surgery as a last resort. I salute these health-care professionals who work tirelessly to seek the causes of disease and advocate true health care, *Naturally*.

This anniversary edition celebrates my recovery and the power of the human spirit to overcome man-made health assaults by entrusting the awesome power of our creator. The following quote by Melodie Beattie says it all!

"Gratitude unlocks the fullness of life—it turns what we have into enough, and more.

It converts denial into acceptance, chaos into order, and confusion into clarity.

It turns problems into gifts, failures into success, the unexpected into perfect timing, and mistakes into important events.

Gratitude makes sense of our past, brings peace for today, and creates a vision for tomorrow."

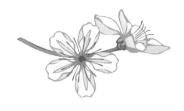

What's Next?

PLENTY! MY WORK HAS JUST BEGUN. I consider it a responsibility to share my knowledge and experiences with as many people as possible—hopefully preventing others from poisoning themselves, as well as continuing to chart the course to recovery for those who are already victims.

I continue to expand my Health Education Travel Programs for "Wholistic Skin & Body Rejuvenation (WSBR)" open to all who choose non-toxic therapies to improve their health and quality of life. (Information is continually updated on my website.)

I'm writing four more books, three courses, and continue to report as a contributing journalist for over eight natural-health publications in the U.S., Canada, and abroad.

I'm developing a line of chemical-free skin care and natural detoxification products based on proven methodologies for rejuvenation.

Additionally, I offer certificated programs for health professionals in destinations around the world; only through teaching

Wholistic Skin and Body Rejuvenation (WSBR®) protocols can we effectively enable others to live healthy in a toxic world and…age without looking or feeling our age.

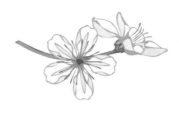

Resources

Testing

Genova Diagnostics (formerly Great Smokies Diagnostic Laboratory)
63 Zillicoa Street, Asheville, NC 28801
(800) 522-4762
Provides the following assessments:
Gastrointestinal, immunology, nutritional, endocrinology, metabolic.

Diagnos-Techs, Inc.
6620 S. 192nd Place, Bldg. J, Kent, WA 98032
(800) 878-3787
Provides the following analyses: Yeast Screens, Digestion Efficiency Panel, GI Pathogen Tests, Melatonin Biorhythm and Challenge Test, NTx Bone Marker Test, Mucosal Barrier Screens, Adrenal Stress Markers, Hormone Panels, Gastrointestinal Health Panel.

Doctor's Data

3755 Illinois Avenue, St. Charles, IL 60174-2420

Tel: (800) 323-2784

Provides the following: Hair Elements Analysis, Whole Blood Elements Analysis, Packed Red Blood Cell Elements Analysis, Urine Elements Analysis, Creatinine Clearance, Urine D-Glucaric and Mercapturic Acid Analyses, Urine and Plasma Amino Acids Analyses, Fecal Toxic Elements, Intestinal Barrier Function Test.

Consulting Clinical and Microbiological Laboratory, Inc.

333 S. W. 5th Avenue, #620-7, Portland, OR 97204

Tel: (503) 222-5279

Provides analyses for infections in the following: respiratory tract, urinary tract, genital tract, gastrointestinal tract.

Meridian Valley Clinical Laboratory

801 SW 16th, Suite 126, Renton, WA 98055

(425) 271-8689

Provides the following analyses: DHEA Screening Blood Lectin Serotypes, Elisa Allergy Tests, Blood Mineral Analysis, Urine Mineral Analysis, Hair Mineral Analysis, Comprehensive Digestive Stool Analysis, Essential Amino Acid Testing, Adrenal Steroids, Parasitology, Essential Fatty Acids, Fractionated Estrogens.

Institute for Parasitic Diseases
3530 E. Indian School Road, Suite 3
Phoenix, AZ 85018
(602) 955-4211
Provides the following analyses: Saliva Tests for Antibodies to Parasites, Clostridium difficile, Helicobacter pylori, and other organisms that may be difficult to detect by stool testing.

Bradford Research Institute
1180 Walnut Avenue, Chula Vista, CA 91911
(800) 227-4473
Provides microscopy services and training as well as referrals to health-care providers utilizing peripheral blood assessments worldwide.

Products

For your convenience, the professional products used and recommended by Gloria Gilbère, as well as her books and E-Guides, may be ordered either by phone toll-free at (888) 352-8175 (U.S. and Canada only) or (208) 255-5252, or online through the Health Matters Store on www.gloriagilbere.com

Note: Some of the professional products may not be listed on the website, but may be ordered directly by phone; ask for details.

**International Association for
Colon Hydrotherapy (I-ACT)**
The governing organization that also provides certification and continuing education for colon therapists. Visit their website at www.i-act.org email at: iact@healthy.net or contact them by calling (210) 366-2888 in San Antonio, Texas USA for a worldwide list of therapists in your region.

The Colon Therapist Network
Provides a membership list of therapist worldwide. Visit their website at www.colontherapist.com.

Consulting with Gloria

To consult with Gloria worldwide by telephone, video cam or at her office in northern Idaho, call **(208) 255-5252** (Monday through Thursday, 8 a.m. to 2 p.m., Pacific time), or log onto her website to *complete forms on the computer, then print, sign in the three indicated areas, and mail along with a recent photo which will not be returned* to:
Gloria Gilbère, N.D., Ph.D.
P.O. Box 1565, Sandpoint, Idaho 83864 USA
   Note: Clients outside of the U.S. may fax their forms to (208) 265-1777.

Gloria's staff does not schedule appointments until all signed forms are received along with a recent photo that will not be returned.

Education

Check Gloria's website at www.gloriagilbere.com for updated information

Educational Travel Programs
Offered twice a year in locations around the world. Check her website for updates.

Wholistic Skin & Body Rejuvenation (WSBR®) Programs
Conducted in world-class hotels, spas, and retreats Individual protocols are designed for each participant, guided by Gloria during the retreat. Check her website for updates.

Certificated WSBR® Programs for Health Professionals
A course to teach natural rejuvenation principles created by Gloria Gilbère. In some states and countries, continuing education credits are available for specific professions. Check her website for updates.

Drugs Classified as Benzodiazepines

The following is a list of some of the drugs classified as benzodiazepines. Benzodiazepines are often produced by different drug companies and thus have different brand names for the same drug.

Generic Name	Brand Name
Alprazolam	Xanax or Kalma
Bromazepam	Lexotan
Clobazam	Frisium
Clonazepam	Rivotril
Clorazepate	Tranxene
Chlordiazepoxide	Librium
Diazepam	Valium, Ducene, or Antenex
Flurazepam	Dalmane
Flunitrazepam	Hypnodorm or Rohypnol
Lorazepam	Ativan
Nitrazepam	Mogadon or Alodorm
Oxazepam	Serax, Serepax, Murelax,, or Alepam
Temazepam	Euhypnos, Nocturne, Normison, Temaze or Temtabs
Triazolam	Halcion

Sleep medications that can have benzo-type side-effects and withdrawal symptoms include, but are not limited to:

Generic Name	Brand Name
Eszopiclone	Lunesta
Zopliclone	Zimovane
Zolpidem	Ambien, Stilnoct
Zaleplon	Sonata

Website Information and Support Groups

Anxiety and Panic Disorders
www.allaboutanxiety.net

Benzodiazepine Symptoms and Withdrawal—
www.benzo.org.uk
www.bcnc.org.uk
www.benzoliberty.com
www.benzodiazepines.cc
www.benzodiazepine.org
www.benzosupport.org
www.drregpeart.org
www.stormloader.com/bettyf

I was

Poisoned

by my body…

Fibromyalgia Coalition International
Support for fibromyalgia, chronic fatigue, and Gulf War syndromes. Membership includes quarterly newletter and discounts at annual conference and other educational forums.
www.fibrocoalition.org

Leaky Gut Syndrome
www.leakygut.co.uk

List of Drugs that Cause
Adverse Psychiatrict Reactions
www.april.org.uk

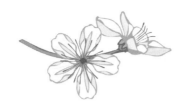

Bibliography

SEVERAL HUNDRED BOOKS, articles, web sites, and manuscripts were reviewed as references for this book. The following is only a representative sampling of those resources.

Allergies Information Center: www.health-n-energy.com

Balch, James F. Dr., and Phyllis A. Balch C.N.C., *Prescription for Nutritional Healing*, Garden City Park, NY: Avery Publishing Group, 1994

BBC News, *Bowel Cancer: The silent killer*, England: Online Network, 1998

Bircher, E. *Food Science for All: New Sunlight Theory of Nutrition.* Health Research Press.

Bland, Jeffrey Dr., *Medical Applications of Clinical Nutrition*, New Canaan, CT: Keats Publishing, 1983

Bland, Jeffrey Dr., *The Inflammatory Disorders,* Washington: Health Comm Seminar Series, 1997

Buchman, Dian Dincin, *Herbal Medicine*, New York, NY: Gramercy Publishing Co., 1980

Canary Connect News, Coralville, IA: Canary Connect Publications, 1998

Carter, Mildred, *Body Reflexology*, West Nyack, NY: Parker Publishing Co., 1983

Cichoke, Anthony Dr., *The Complete Book of Enzyme Therapy,* Garden City Park, NY: Avery Publishing Group, 1999

Crook, William Dr., *The Yeast Connection*, New York, NY: Vintage Books, 1986

The Drug and Natural Medicine Advisor, Richmond, VA: Time Life Custom Publishing, 1997

Dumke, Nicolette, *Allergy Cooking with Ease*, Lancaster, PA: Starburst Publishers, 1992

Dumke, Nicolette, *5 Years without Food, The Food Allergy Survival Guide*, Louisville, CO: Adapt Books, 1997

Effects of Whole Live Foods on (SOD) Deficiency in 10 Adult Humans, Conducted by Dr. Peter Rothschild, M.D., Ph.D., et al. Testing by Smith-Kline Bio-Science, Honolulu, HI. Antioxidant enzymes supplied by Biotec Food, HI. Courtesy of AgriGeneic Food Corp. Huntington Beach, CA

Ewing, W.N. and D.J.A. Cole, *The Living Gut*, England: Redwood Books, 1994

Gittleman, Ann Louise, *Guess What Came to Dinner—Parasites and your Health*, Garden City Park, NY: Avery Publishing Group, 1993

Golan, Ralph Dr., *Optimal Wellness*, New York, NY: Ballantine Books, 1995

Golos, Natalie, and Golos Frances Golbitz, *If This is Tuesday, It Must be Chicken*, New Canaan, CT: Keats Publishing, 1983

Gray, Robert, *The Colon Health Handbook,* Reno, NV: Emerald Publishing, 1991

Haas, Elson Dr., *Staying Healthy with the Seasons*, Berkeley, CA: Celestial Arts, 1981

Hagiwara, Yoshihide. *Green Barley Essence: A Surprising Source of Health*. Tokyo, Japan: Association of Green and Health Distributors, 1981.

Heimlich, Jane, *What Your Doctor Won't Tell You*, New York, NY: Harper Perennial, 1990

Heinerman, John, *Heinerman's Encyclopedia of Healing Juices*, West Nyack, NY: Parker Publishing Company, 1994

Jamison, Alcinous Dr., *Intestinal Ills*, New York, NY: Chas. Tyrrell M.D., 1917

Jensen, Bernard Dr., *Tissue Cleansing Through Bowel Managment*, Escondido, CA: Bernard Jensen Enterprises, 1981.

Kellogg, John Harvey Dr., *Colon Hygiene*, Battle Creek, MI: Modern Medicine Publishing Co., 1923

Kenton, L. and Kenton, S., *Raw Energy*, London: Century Publishing, 1984

Ley, Beth, *Castor Oil: Its Healing Properties*, Aliso Viejo, CA: BL Publications, 1989

Lipski, Elizabeth, *Digestive Wellness*, New Canaan, CT: Keats Publishing, 1996

Loes, Michael Dr., and Steinman, David M.A., *The Aspirin Alternative,* Topanga, CA: Freedom Press, 1999

Loomis, Howard Dr., Enzymes, *The Key to Health*, Madison WI: 21st Century Nutrition Publication, 1999

Lopez, D.A. Dr., and Williams, R.M. Dr., Miehlke, K. Dr., *Enzymes: The Fountain of Life*, Charleston, SC: The Neville Press, 1994

Losenvold, Lloyd Dr., *Can a Gluten-Free Diet Help?*, New Canaan, CT: Keats Publishing, 1992

Lust, John, *Drink Your Troubles Away,* New York, NY: Benedict Lust Publications, 1967

The Merck Manual of Medical Information, Whitehouse Station, N.J: Merck Research Laboratories, 1997

McWilliams, Peter and Roger, John, *You Can't Afford the Luxury of a Negative Thought*, Los Angeles, CA: Prelude Press, 1988

Meyerowitz, S. *Wheat Grass: Nature's Finest Medicine.* Book Publishing Co., Summertown, TN. 1999

Millard, F.P. Dr., and Walmsley, A.G. Dr., *Applied Anatomy of the Lymphatics*, Mokelumne Hill, CA: Health Research, 1964

MFA Collection, Coeur d'Alene, ID: MAST Enterprises, 1986

MuCos, *Oral Enzymes*, Germany: Mucos Pharma Gmbh & Co., 1992

Physicians' Desk Reference, 50th Edition, 1996

Robinson, Arthur, "Living Foods and Cancer," *Hippocrates Newsletter*, March, 1984.

Rogers, Sherry Dr., *You Are What You Ate*, Syracuse, NY: Prestige Publishing, 1997

Rogers, Sherry Dr., *The E.I. Syndrome*, Syracuse, NY: Prestige Publishers, 1986

Rogers, Sherry Dr., *Wellness Against All Odds*, Syracuse, NY: Prestige Publishing, 1994

Schmidt, Michael A., Smith, Lendon H., Sehnert, Keith W., Beyond Antibiotics, *50 (or so) Ways to Boost Immunity and Avoid Antibiotics*, Berkeley, CA: North Atlantic Books, 1993

Shabert, Judy Dr., and Ehrlich, Nancy, *The Ultimate Nutrient Glutamine*, Garden City Park, NY: Avery Publishing Group, 1994

Special Report: *Aloe Vera & You*, Orlando, FL: Pinnacle Printing, 1994

Stoll, Walt Dr., *Saving Yourself from the Disease-Care Crisis*, Panama City, FL: 1996

Tenney, Louise M.H., *Colon Health*, Pleasant Grove, UT: Woodland Publishing, 1998

Thie, John, *Touch for Health*, Marina del Ray, CA: DeVorss and Company, 1995.

Truss, Orian Dr., *The Missing Diagnosis*, Birmingham, Al: The Missing Diagnosis, Inc., 1983

United States Pharmacopeia The, Rockville, MD: United States Pharmacopeial Convention, 1995

Van der Hulst, RRWJ, *Glutamine, an essential nutrient for the gut*, University of Maastricht, Germany: 1996

Walker, Norman Dr., *Colon Health*, Prescott, AZ: Norwalk Press, 1995

Weinberger, Stanley C.M.T., *Parasites—An Epidemic in Disguise*, Larkspur, CA: Healing Within, 1993

Weiss, Jennifer N.D., and Burnett Vena N.D., *Colon Cleansing, The Best-Kept Secret*, Auburn, CA: The Sunshine Company, 1989

Wigmore, Ann, *The Wheatgrass Book*, Garden City Park, NY: Avery Publishing Group, 1985

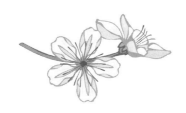

Index

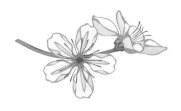

About the Author

GLORIA GILBÈRE IS A TRADITIONAL NATUROPATH, homeopath, doctor of natural health, eco-ergonomist, environmental health consultant, and internationally renowned for her wholistic skin and body rejuvenation (WSBR®) programs. Her professional affiliations include, but are not limited to:

Member—
   American Academy of Environmental Medicine
   American Naturopathic Medical Association
   National Coalition for Natural Health
   American Association of Nutritional Consultants
   American Society of Safety Engineers (R)

Diplomate—Academy of Homeopathy

Advisory Board—
   Vista Magazine of Canada
   Anxiety & Panic Attack Resource Center

Natural Body Cures

Leaky Gut Syndrome Support Center (U.K.)

Board Member—Fibromyalgia Coalition Int'l

Associate Editor —*Total Health* Magazine

Adjunct Professor—

Clayton College of Natural Health

She is founder and director of the international consulting consortium, Global Integrated Health, a health care consulting firm made-up of a network of highly trained and specialized naturopaths, integrative medical doctors and professionals in varied modalities of natural and integrative health. These professionals provide consulting and referral services to clients worldwide.

Gloria maintains a private global practice based in northern Idaho. Her services include clinical work, telephone consultation (nationally and internationally) with clients, researchers, and physicians.

She teaches, lectures and consults worldwide, is a prominent health journalist and medical researcher, and has written over 400 articles for newspapers, health magazines and trade journals.

She is a sought-after guest on radio, television, professional conferences and educational institutions, as well as talk-show host of *Your Health Matters*, heard weekly on www.healthylife.net internet radio.

Gloria is a keynote presenter and conducts seminars on varied disciplines of wholistic health, multiple allergic response syndrome (MARS), leaky gut syndrome (LGS), chemically induced immune system disorders, and has earned international acclaim for her *Wholistic Skin & Body Rejuvenation (WSBR®) Programs.* Her work has taken her throughout the U.S. and more than 30 countries.

She is internationally respected as a natural medicine researcher and an authoritative influence in the discovery of the causes, effects and natural solutions for leaky gut syndrome and chemically induced immune system disorders.

As a consultant, educator, and trainer in preventive health care, environmental color psychology, and EcoErgonomics, her client list includes Fortune 500 companies, universities, hospitals, health-care organizations, government agencies, school districts, corporations, small businesses, and professional associations.

For information regarding her services, speaking engagements and interviews:

Voice—(208) 255-5252 (Monday through Thursday Pacific Standard Time, U.S.)

Fax—(208) 265-1777

Email—gloria@gloriagilbere.com

Visit her website at—www.gloriagilbere.com

Write—Gloria Gilbère, N.D., Ph.D.

P.O. Box 1565, Sandpoint, Idaho 83864 USA